July, 1988

To Scott and Mary,

With ~~thanks~~ and best wishes — John Ireson

The WAY of LIFE

The WAY of LIFE

Macrobiotics and The Spirit of Christianity

The Seven Principles of The Infinite Universe
Interpreted in the Language and Imagery of the Bible

by The Rev. John Ineson

Drawings by Ted Keller

Japan Publications, Inc.

Published by JAPAN PUBLICATIONS, INC., Tokyo & New York

Distributors:
UNITED STATES: *Kodansha International/USA, Ltd., through Harper & Row, Publishers, Inc., 10 East 53rd Street, New York, N.Y. 10022.* SOUTH AMERICA: *Harper & Row, Publishers, Inc., International Department.* CANADA: *Fitzhenry & Whiteside Ltd., 195 Allstate Parkway, Markham, Ontario, L3R 4T8.* MEXICO & CENTRAL AMERICA: *HARLA S. A. de C. V., Apartado 30-546, Mexico 4, D. F.* BRITISH ISLES: *International Book Distributors Ltd., 66 Wood Lane End, Hemel Hempstead, Herts HP2 4RG.* EUROPEAN CONTINENT: *Fleetbooks, S. A., c/o Feffer and Simons (Nederland) B. V., Rijnkade 170, 1382 GT Weesp, The Netherlands.* AUSTRALIA & NEW ZEALAND: *Bookwise International, 1 Jeanes Street, Beverley, South Australia 5007.* THE FAR EAST & JAPAN: *Japan Publications Trading Co., Ltd., 1-2-1, Sarugaku-cho, Chiyoda-ku, Tokyo 101.*

First edition: April 1986

LCCC No. 85-080539
ISBN 0-87040-635-3

Printed in U.S.A.

To Anna, Ted, Susan, and the everchanging cast of that unique drama:

THE WAY OF LIFE CENTER

"The are two ways: the way of life and the way of death."
The Didaché, or *Teaching of the Twelve Apostles*

". . . I have set before you life and death, blessing and curse; therefore choose life . . . for that means life to you and length of days." (Deuteronomy 30 : 19, 20)

Contents

Acknowledgments

Dictionaries include the connotation of gratitude in the definition of "acknowledge," but not until the fourth or fifth definition. I want it to be clear that my gratitude is not only implied in acknowledgment but that acknowledgment is implied in my abounding gratitude.

Above all I am grateful for being in this place at this turning point in human history and wish to acknowledge the part my parents, grandparents, and ancestors had and continue to have in my being here as who I am.

Heartfelt gratitude also encompasses the following:

All those who bade my spirit, "Rise!" by both their love and their fear of loving.

Anna, live-in editor, wife, counselor, macrobiotic cook and my prime reason for being (not necessarily in that order).

My daughters, Beth and Amy, whose growth in wisdom, stature, and Grace has provided nineteen years of joy-filled fascination plus a lot of corny jokes.

Ted Keller, whose drawings grace this volume and whose life is an ongoing demonstration of the manifestation of the Grace of God in macrobiotics.

Ed Esko, whose suggestion it was that I write this book; Michio Kushi, whose power to inspire is inestimable, and who made publication of this book possible.

Jamie Tietjen, computer whiz, who appeared at my door, lived in my house and gathered oddly contrived files into a publishable manuscript, thus saving me from unspeakable anxieties.

Parishioners of St. Andrew's Episcopal Church, Newcastle, Maine, whose patience with my busy schedule and whose enthusiasm in our ministry together is whole food for the inner being.

The hundreds of writers whose works have been inwardly digested over the years, portions of whose discoveries have been quoted in this book by permission as noted below:

Science 82. November edition, Copyright © 1982, The American Association for the Advancement of Science.

Seven Basic Macrobiotic Principles. Published by The Grain and Salt Society.

The Silence of Jesus. Copyright © 1983, Doubleday Canada, Ltd., by permission of Fortress Press.

The Witness. Vol. 68, No. 1, Copyright © 1985, The Witness.

Virgil: The Georgics. Copyright © 1982 L. P. Wilkinson, by permission of Penguin Books, Ltd.

You are All Sanpaku. Copyright © 1965, University Books, Inc., by permission of Citadel Press.

Zen Macrobiotics. Copyright © 1965, Ohsawa Foundation, Inc., by permission of George Ohsawa Macrobiotic Foundation.

Introduction

One morning at daybreak Aristotle was walking the shore of the Mediterranean, contemplating the universe, when he spied a figure in the distance. The person appeared to be running a short distance from the water's edge to the sand and back again. As the distance between them grew shorter Aristotle could see that it was the village madman, and he was carrying something from the water and back again. Soon he saw what was going on; the man had a small cup and was taking water from the sea and pouring it in a hole he had dug in the sand. After the usual pleasantries, Aristotle asked him what he was doing. "I'm going to empty the sea into this hole, here, and I'll be able to see the beautiful green and blue sand that covers the floor of the sea and shines up through the water," the madman explained. "You'll never get the whole Mediterranean in that little hole," Aristotle responded, pointing to the small depression the man had dug. The madman looked at him quizzically and asked, "What are you doing walking the beach so early in the day?" "I am a philosopher," Aristotle replied, "and I am contemplating the universe." The madman came closer and, putting a finger to Aristotle's temple, said, "You'll never get the whole universe in that little head!"

From earliest times human beings have been trying to get the whole universe in our little heads, to explain life's mysteries, to devise a thought structure upon which answers could be hung. This striving has resulted in major philosophical movements, folk wisdom, complex ceremonies, arcane rituals, every conceivable manner of divination, and methods of which we have not conceived but that have been revealed through archaeological excavation. Each one of us has built a system of understanding to advise us when we confront life's dilemmas. Sometimes our system agrees with the system of others to the extent that we can meet in groups to celebrate our system and to reinforce each others' beliefs.

There are those who believe that they have the answers—all the answers. They are the ones whom C. S. Lewis describes as believing that they have balanced the right hand and left hand pages of the ledger of reality and can "close the books" satisfied that the answers balance the questions. Several years ago there was a proliferation of bumper stickers displayed by such people which said, "I FOUND IT!" In a typically American response there then appeared bumper stickers proclaiming, "I NEVER LOST IT!"

At the other end of the spectrum are those who have abandoned the search for intellectually appealing answers and hold the view that, ultimately, we do not know, that at the deepest level of being, the answer to "know thyself" is that each of us is "I don't know."

Both of these views have found adherents in major religions and philosophical systems. However, both of these views co-exist today in the major religion of the West, Christianity. Within the Christian tradition exists and extraordinarily wide interpretation of what has traditionally been called "the faith once delivered to the saints." The I FOUND IT people are part of the born again movement. The I DON'T KNOW adherents are of equally ancient origins and are found in monasteries, convents, and on the streets wherever the tradition of the 14th Century English mystical treatise *The Cloud of Unknowing* finds validation.

Most of us fall somewhere between those who know and those who know they do not. We feel certain about some things and are at a loss to explain satisfactorily other facets of the jewel we call life. Even those who identify themselves as believers encounter explanations within their official belief system in which they just cannot believe. The whole realm of scientific thought has, over the years, come to be seen as antagonistic to religion because science offers explanations for things which had been considered the realm of divine activity beyond our understanding. The workings of many mysteries of this universe still may be placed under the heading, "God Only Knows." This is a "God in the gaps" theology which sooner or later must shrink to oblivion as more and more mysteries are demystified through scientific discovery. The "God in the gaps" stance is made on shaky and diminishing ground. Yet, the village madman was right. We cannot get the whole universe into our little heads.

Despite the gallons of ink spilled by theologians throughout the ages, the Christian tradition sides more closely with the madman's estimation of Aristotle's endeavors than with the notion that all the answers can be found, codified, and described in a *summa theologica*. Early attempts to find salvation through knowledge were branded heresy by the young Church and Gnosticism's view of Jesus as divine messenger boy was given wide berth by Church councils and theologians. The reasons are many why an almost anti-intellectual theme plays through Church history, and, in spite of the fact that mighty intellects have been counted in her ranks weighty works produced, and universities founded and supported by her, the underlying understanding is that at the heart of the Church's teaching lies a secret, a mystery. In the Epistle to the Colossians Paul states that it is his ministry "to announce the secret hidden for long ages," (1:26), but when he announces this secret, the secret turns out to be a truly phenomenal mystery: "The secret is this: Christ is in you, your hope of a glory to come," (1:27b). Somehow the answer to the *mysterium tremendum* is another mystery —union of the believer with the Christ. How? In what way? The answer to that is another mystery, the mystery of faith, that which "gives substance to our hopes, and makes us certain of realities we do not see," (Hebrews 11:1). "For through faith you are all sons of God in union with Christ Jesus," (Galatians 3:26).

That this faith and this union with the Christ is possible lies at the heart of the Good News. All cognitive theories and intellectual speculation must be seen as attempts by finite aspects of human nature to grasp the infinite. Indeed, it is a demonstration of incredible arrogance even to imply that we can get the whole universe in our little heads, but, implications notwithstanding, we search; we knock at doors in hope that this time they will open and that they will ultimately lead us to that door which stands at Eden's East gate—the one which leads to the tree of life.

Many Westerners come to the macrobiotic way of life out of a Christian tradition which has historically rejected contact with the philosophy of the East. This exclusivity is understandable when the history of the development of Christianity is considered. Judaism clung tenaciously to its unique monotheism in the face of attractive polytheistic religions throughout the era of its occupation of the promised land and during contact with Graeco-Roman religions. In addition to inheriting this bias, early Christianity found itself spreading into the world of Zoroastrianism and Greek mystery cults. The helenizing influence sought to turn Jesus' eminently practical and profoundly simple religion of love and new life into a complex philosophical system where, as in Greek thought, reason ruled. Over the centuries the Church has formulated creeds, canon law, and a myriad of defenses in an attempt to keep the faith of the early Church intact. This stance was bred of necessity, but it has its unfortunate side: the Church, in its desire to exclude obvious heresy, has tended to insulate itself from other interpretations of commonly held basic truths.

The Christian macrobiotic is often ill-prepared to deal with the concepts, folk wisdom, and philosophy found in macrobiotic literature. This fact places no one at fault, but is purely the function of the influence of the Christian movement and scientific bias on Western culture. The philosophical basis of macrobiotics and its interpretation is clear and concise. However, the emphasis on experiential and intuitive evidence requires, in many cases, more flexibility than is found in many Westerners who are exposed to macrobiotic theory. Brief self reflection is all that is required to realize how much every life is lived on a basis grounded in experience and intuition. The issue of Eastern philosophical rhetoric, however, raises an even more serious impediment to those nurtured in the Christian tradition. Terms such as Heaven's Force, Yin and Yang, Celestial Influence, Earth's Force, and astrological signs may well be associated with Eastern religions, geomancy, and astrology. Where, in Christian rhetoric, do these concepts find meaning? Is macrobiotics a religion?

The Didache, meaning "teaching," an early Christian document attributed to the Apostles, begins with the words, "There are two ways: the way of life and the way of death." Macrobiotics is not a religion. It is a way of life which has as its cornerstone *The Seven Universal Principles of The Infinite Universe,* a statement of the most basic truths concerning the nature of the "way of life." Their interpretation has given rise to a growing corpus of macrobiotic literature.

Most of this literature has arisen from the cultural milieu of the Orient, incorporating Eastern philosophy and understandings, many of which are truly foreign to readers in the West. However, these principles are universal and can be interpreted in the language and thought forms of any culture.

There has been no single influence more pervasive in shaping the thinking of the West than Christianity. The language and thought forms of the West find their roots in the Christian tradition or in reaction to the Christian tradition. At the heart of Christianity are universal truths recognizable in all world religions. Among these truths are the seven universal principles of macrobiotic philosophy and all which they imply. The language of the religion of the West is a suitable vehicle for interpreting the wisdom of the principles rediscovered in the East.

No one person can speak for Christianity today. Two thousand years of doctrinal, liturgical, and canonical evolution has resulted in "Found Its," "Never Lost Its," fundamentalists, liberals, conservatives, mystics, humanists, and a host of interpreters who represent, nonetheless, the Church today. Even within a single tradition or denomination one may find all of the above represented. Therefore, we are driven back to a time when the message of love, forgiveness, and union with the divine through faith seemed simpler if only by virtue of having fewer interpreters. The faith of the early Church is presented to us in the writings of the New Testament. These writings cover a period of some seventy years from the decade of the 50's, when Paul wrote his epistles, to about A.D. 120, when the writings of John were penned. Scholars disagree on dates as a matter of course, it seems, so these dates should be used as approximations at best.

These writings represent a sort of frozen tradition of the faith of the Church at the time that they were written. They, too, represent a wide diversity of interpretation and reflect disagreement within the ranks of believers, but in studying them one can certainly grasp the spirit of Christianity as it spread like sparks through the stubble into a world populated by a myriad of beliefs. The Bible, in particular the New Testament, will, therefore, be used as our common reference point as we seek to interpret the Seven Universal Principles in the language of the religion of the West. In so doing perhaps we can get a little more of this universe into our little heads.

PART I

The Seven Principles of The Infinite Universe

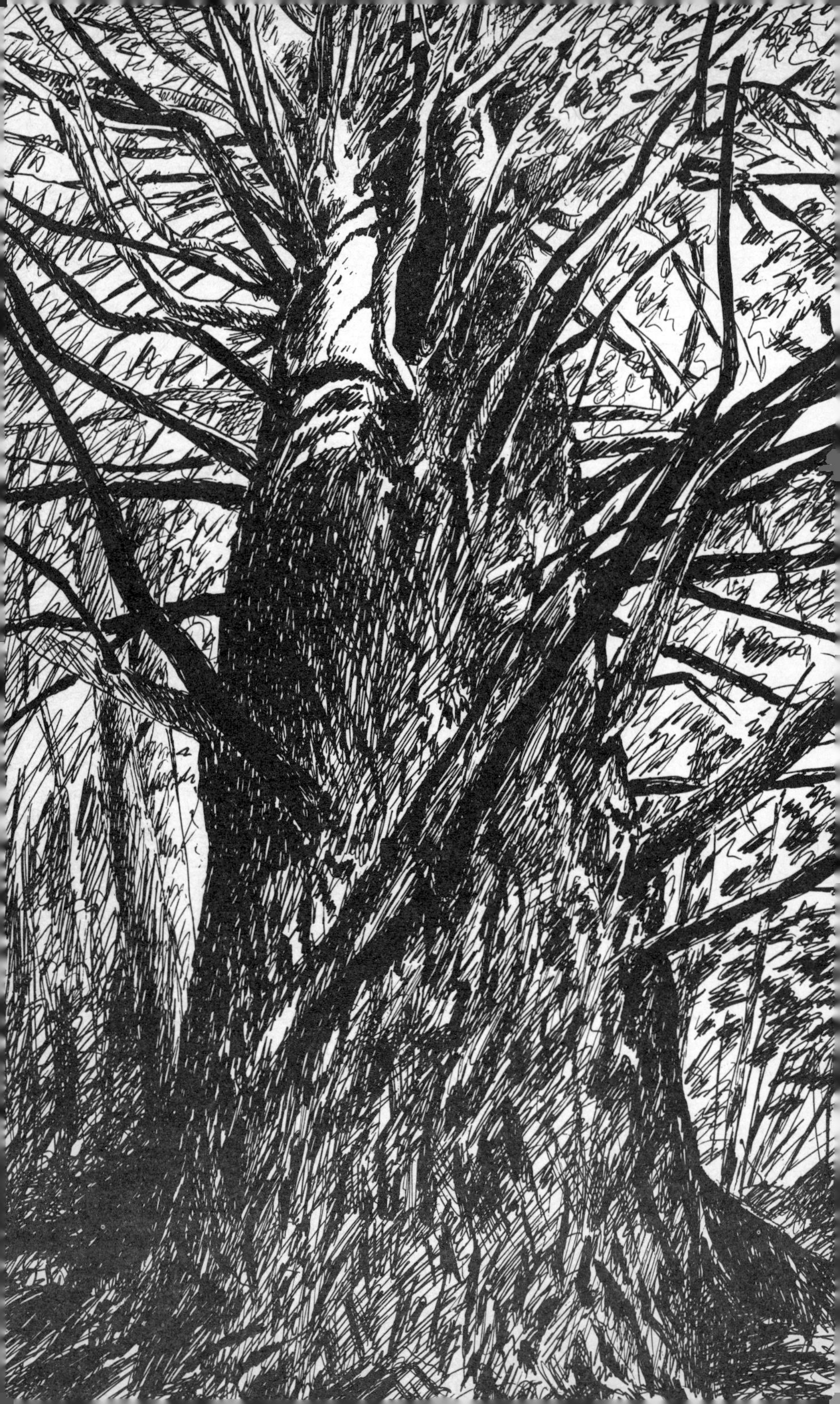

Chapter 1

Everything is a Differentiation of One Infinity

"The Lord, our God, is one."
(Deuteronomy 6:4; Mark 12:29)

ON THE 50TH WEDDING ANNIVERSARY of my paternal grandparents, my grandfather, Charles Edward, looked at his wife Jessie Dean, and said, "It's most beautiful, Jessie, once there were only two of us!" They were surrounded by thirty six direct descendants and an even greater number of in-laws, friends and acquaintances drawn to the celebration of the day 50 years before when, indeed, there were only two. His exclamation has taken on even greater significance over the many intervening years, and it is one which I have treasured. To our limited view, the growth of family members does seem to be an endless, expanding cycle of birth, growth, and death. As a young only child, I was impressed mightily by that anniversary gathering of extended family.

One creative energy lies behind all we perceive, one Word issuing from the mouth of infinity, echoing through the vast abyss of interstellar space. The breath on which this Word is carried creates all that is and sweeps into manifestation not only us and our world but the very power to perceive it. Everything is a differentiation of this one infinity. The truth of the One Behind the Many lies at the heart of Judaism, Christianity,

Islam, native American spirituality, Taoism, and a host of understandings with too few adherents to be classified as major religions.

One of the most ancient statements of this truth is found in the book of Deuteronomy. This book was discovered in the temple at Jerusalem during the reign of Josiah, King of Judah from 640 to 609 B.C. Scholars believe that it was written during the reign of Manasseh, holder of the same office earlier in that century. Ideas which appear in ancient writings are usually a long time in development and are part of an oral tradition for many years before being penned. "Hear, O Israel, the Lord our God, the Lord is One," (Deuteronomy 6:4). This is an Old Testament maxim which set apart the children of Israel from their polytheistic neighbors. Manifestations of Canaanite polytheism, from household idols to temple prostitution, so galvanized the zeal of the monotheistic Hebrews that wheels of exclusivity were set in motion which still turn today in both Judaism and Christianity. The words from Deuteronomy are found on the lips of Jesus in Mark's gospel as a preamble to what has come to be called The Summary of The Law: the admonition to love God and to love our neighbor as ourself. Paul echoes the theme in his statement "There is no God but one . . . for us there is one God, the Father, from whom all being comes, towards whom we move," (1 Corinthians 8:4, 6). He states the same truth in the poetry of 1 Corinthians 12:4–11: "There are varieties of Gifts, but the same Spirit."

For beings who have a beginning and an end to contemplate "beginninglessness" and endlessness is an impossibility of the first order, and, yet, perhaps the need to do this is one of the major vitalizing influences of the human condition. Gerhard Tersteegen said, "A comprehended God is no God at all," and, although we may understand this in our heads, our hearts are restless in the search for comprehension. St. Augustine expressed this restlessness, "My heart is restless until it finds its rest in Thee." I can remember as a young boy having to stop thinking about infinity because it made me dizzy. I would imagine leaving earth and going through outer space with the awareness that there was no end to it. When my cognitive faculties, which are with beginning and end, came face to face with the reality of endlessness the dizziness would set in. The lifelong search and the always ensuing dizziness are bound up in the impossibility of searching for the One who "dwells in light inaccessible to mortal eyes," (1 Timothy 6: 16; 1 Corinthians 13: 8).

There was no question in the minds of early Christian believers that there was only one God. The roots which fed the fast-branching Church were Jewish; her Lord and Master was raised a Jew; the Father was One and Jesus was one with the Father extending his interpretation of this unity to all who followed his way of life, "May they all be one: as thou, Father, art in me and I in thee, so also may they be in us that the world may believe that thou didst send me. The glory which thou gavest me I have given to them, that they may be one, as we are one; I in them and thou in me, may they be perfectly one," (John 17: 21–23). John reports these words of Jesus and they represent the faith of the Church at the time they were written.

Strict definitions of the faith were necessitated as other interpretations arose among the ranks of heretics, those who stressed one aspect of the truth to the exclusion of others. The Church councils were assembled to debate these heresies and, as a result, statements of faith or creeds were drawn up to define what was considered orthodox belief. A list of heresies reads like a catalogue of tongue-twisters: Monophysitism, Monothelitism, Eutychians, Nestorians, Antiochenes, Ebionites, Arians, Apollinarians, Sabellians. The most widely recognized creed, still in use today in Western Christianity, bears a full title which sounds as if it takes a tongue-twister to judge a tongue-twister: The Nicaeano-Constantinopolitan Creed. The creed was adopted in the year 325 at the Council of Nicaea and was confirmed as orthodox at the Council of Constantinople in 381. It begins with the words "We believe in one God."

Even the heretics held the basic truth of monotheism. Their heresies lay in just how this one God became incarnate in the person of Jesus and the nature of the relationship between Father, Son, and Holy Spirit. The Council of Smirnium in 357, adopted a creed called by Hilary of Poitiers "The Blasphemy of Smirnium," because it incorporated the ideas of the heresy of Arianism which denied the true divinity of Jesus Christ. This position was overcorrected by another heresy propounded by Apollinarius, Bishop of Laodicea, who died in 392 and emphasized the divinity of Jesus at the expense of his full manhood. However, "The Blasphemy" begins with the undisputed words, "It is agreed that there is one God." The Dated Creed of 359 elaborates somewhat on the statement with the words, "We believe in one God, the only and the true God."

"God is one," says Meister Eckhart, the late 13th to early 14th century German Dominican mystic, "and lives within his own pure being which contains nothing else. He himself is a pure presence in which there is neither this nor that, because what is in God is God!" Chuang Tzu, writing from a vastly different cultural and religious ethos describes the viewpoint of the Simple Man as "one at which this and that, yes and no, appear still in a state of nondistinction. From it only Infinity is to be seen, which is neither this nor that, nor yes nor no. To see all in the yet undifferentiated primordial unity, or from such a distance that all melts into one, this is true intelligence."

Those of us raised with the notion that true intelligence is defined by achieving some score over one hundred on the Stanford-Binet Intelligence Quotient Test may find a definition embodying intuitive and mystical qualities difficult to accept. The idea of intelligence being restricted to cognitive faculties is far more a product of the age of reason than it is a long held view. To the ancients, intelligence was more than intellectual capacity, just as perception was not limited to that of the five senses. In many ways, we have come to think of ourselves as far more limited beings than did our forebears. Reasons for this reflect the effects of the Copernican revolution and the ability of today's science to measure the micro and macrocosm. Copernicus declared that the sun does not revolve around us; that in fact the case is just the opposite. We are not the center of the universe. What a profound effect on the human consciousness that pronouncement must have had! We now know that it takes light one hundred thousand years just to cross our galaxy, and that our galaxy is only one of billions. We are no more than specks on a speck!

One would expect that a theology which expounds the coming of the Creator into creation as a human being would be phenomenally compelling because of its elevation of human nature. But, as the scientific bias has gained ascendancy, the attraction of Christianity seems to be diminishing. A possible reason for this bears directly on the subject of this chapter: when we lose the viewpoint of Chuang Tzu's Simple Man, the viewpoint of all saints and sages, we become so caught up in "this and that" that the One from whom "this and that" flow becomes inaccessible, indeed.

How do we recover the "eyes to see and the ears to hear" which Jesus tells us are necessary to know the truth which sets us free from a world limited to this and that?

Both the implicit monotheism of macrobiotics and the explicit belief in one God in Christianity stand as a common cornerstone on which both structures depend. Not only is there no difference between the "infinite One" of macrobiotics and the One God of Christianity, but both share the truth that our hearts are restless until they find their rest in that One (to paraphrase Augustine). Both Christianity and macrobiotics illuminate a way to recover our sight, our hearing, our true intelligence, an opportunity to see face to face what we now only "see through a glass darkly," (1 Corinthians 13:12). In that famous passage from 1 Corinthians Paul says, "the partial vanishes when wholeness comes." The micro view vanishes when the macro view appears. Seeing face to face is the viewpoint of Chuang Tzu's Simple Man. It is the beatific vision; it is the highest level of judgment; it makes our joy full.

The "spiral of creation" so prevalent in macrobiotic literature describes the course of material and physical manifestation through ever-tightening turns from the Infinite One to the animal kingdom. Increasingly more complex phenomena are traced from the first arising of polarity to vibration to preatomic particles, to elements, to vegetable matter to the animal kingdom. The spiral does not stop there. The most complex beings in the animal kingdom, those whom Jerome Canty describes as being at "the crack of the whip," begin the returning course to the One Infinity. The purpose of our being is to complete the round trip and to do it consciously. A multitude of spiritual disciplines, self-help techniques, and philosophical understandings point to this purpose as well. Both the Christian religion and the macrobiotic way of life, which complements any religious system, point to the true direction of life's journey. Both also hold that to take responsibility for this return trip is the task to which each of us is assigned by this loving universe. Experience informs us "You must work out your own salvation with fear and trembling," (Philippians 2:12), not that we must be fearful but that this is a business to be taken seriously; it is a call to personal responsibility; it is a reminder that until we are born again into a realization of the reality of the spiritual realm there is no salvation from being caught up in the realm of "this and that." These are not new words or new concepts. Anyone who has been led to the active search for wider horizons, attended Church, read the works of saints and sages, or sought the truth has heard this all before.

What is it that keeps us from that point of balance where the Father and we are perceived to be one? Among other things it is the anesthesia of repetition. The stories the Church holds dear and repeats season after liturgical season, the passages from scripture mocked by Madison Avenue have become too familiar. Aphorisms, truisms, sound parental advice, all have bombarded us until we are deaf to their truths. Studies done on change of attitudes point to the necessity of dissonance before the change can be effected. The dissonance may be physical, emotional, psychological, or spiritual and come any number of sources such as a change of job, death of a loved one, manifestation of a life-threatening disease, radical change in lifestyle whether voluntary or involuntary, or any other event which could be described as an important life change. The anesthesia wears off as soon as we are shaken up. Otherwise we are like the man in this old Sufi story:

Alexandria, in Egypt, was a great center of learning. The library there was reputed to have 750,000 scrolls covering Eastern and Western philosophical traditions. Scientific treatises and esoteric knowledge were stored away in the archives. In the second Century, Alexandrine theology was a potent force in shaping the theology of the Church. The library was destroyed in a series of lootings and burnings carried out by invading forces who sought to strike at the heart of one of the vivifying influences in this great city. During one such book-burning a bystander rushed forward, tucked what was left of one of the scrolls in his robes and hurried home with his prize. Upon reading the manuscript he discovered that it described the whereabouts of a stone which would transmute any metal it touched to gold. His heart beat faster. Here was the answer to his poverty, his dreams of wealth, an escape from the squalor in which he lived.

Immediately he sold what few things he had and made for the place where this stone lay, the shore of the Black Sea. Anyone finding this stone would recognize it upon picking it up, the manuscript had explained; it was warm to the touch. His first night was spent in wakeful anticipation, and dawn found him by the water's edge. But how to be sure that the millions of stones would be handled only once? The perfect plan came to him. He would throw each stone tested into the water and, thus, not encounter it again as he made his way along the shore. All day he picked up stones, tested them and tossed them into the sea. All the next day he would pick up a stone—cold—throw into the water—pick up a stone—cold—throw into the water—pick up a stone—cold—throw into the water. For days upon days he did this, from sun-up to sunset, by moonlight, in the rain. This went on for months and then one day he picked up a stone and it was warm! He threw it far out into the sea.

This man lives in each of us. For years we search for the stone which will transmute our shallow understanding into the deep riches of wisdom. For years we handle what could be the stone whose inner warmth identifies it as able to bestow those riches. How many times have we had it in our hands only to throw it away out of habit? How many times have stormy situations, life's dissonances, washed it back upon our shore only to be discarded again? In fact, this stone is with us every moment in the omnipresence of the infinite One: "He is not far from each one of us, for in Him we live and move and have our being," (Acts 17:28). There is no place we can go apart from this presence: "Where can I escape from thy spirit? Where can I flee from thy presence? If I climb up to heaven, thou art there; if I make my bed in Sheol, again I find thee. If I take my flight to the frontiers of the morning or dwell at the limit of the western sea, even there thy hand will meet me and thy right hand will hold me fast," (Psalm 139:7–10); and again, "For I am convinced that there is nothing in death or life, in the realm of spirits or superhuman powers, in the world as it is or the world as it shall be, in the forces of the universe, in heights or depths—nothing in all creation that can separate us from the love of God in Christ Jesus our Lord," (Romans 8:38, 39).

When Jesus is quoted as saying, "For you have one father and he is in heaven," (Matthew 23:9) and "My father and I are one," (John 10:30) the gospel writers are describing the place in our consciousness where the stone of our salvation may be found. Were this truth lived moment to moment there would be no need to read on nor to write on. There is a door deep in our being behind which this truth lives and from under which issues a great light. How often we knock at it, try to shoulder it open, or attempt to pick the lock! The door is unlocked and the handle is only on one side, the side at which we stand.

Perhaps our resistance to living the truth of the unity of creation lies in a basic distrust of the nature of the universe. Is the universe without purpose, a chance happening which commingles the good and the bad, the grotesque with the beautiful in a capricious and careless tragi-comic production? Or is it an orderly interplay of divine energy emanating from One source and throughout which that source may be experienced and identified as endlessly loving and sustaining? Are the things in which we participate mere chance happenings perpetrated by a heartless cosmic economy, or are our life experiences drawn to us, given to us for our learning and growth as we inexorably move toward the infinite One from whose bosom we came? The Biblical record solidly supports the latter in both cases, and although the possibility of the former is raised it is done so only as a vehicle to transport the truth of a loving infinity differentiating into a creation which is good and in which the only ultimate power is that of good. The books of the Bible are a record of the One differentiating into one thousand years of history in which the specifics of that differentiation, the historical events, are seen as inseparable from that One. In the language of the Bible, Holy Scripture is the story of God at work in history among his chosen people, chosen in that they, of all people known to them, recognize His fatherhood. For the people of the Bible the creator is forever at work in "this and that" and the purpose of creation is best seen in the interpretation of historical events. The God of the Bible is a God of history.

Later theological development prompted by the influence of Greek philosophy upon the practical and pragmatic Hebrew theology has almost erased the memory of the Old Testament roots of Christian understanding. If we were to ask a Hebrew of Old Testament times what a chair is we would be told that it is something to sit on. If we were to ask the same question of a Greek philosopher we would receive a discourse on "chairness." When the practical is compared with the speculative in theology we behold a god of history on one hand and, on the other, a god best understood not in terms of what he does but rather by what he is.

The trinitarian controversy (how God can be one substance and three persons) dominated the theological life of the early Church, gave rise to the tongue-twisters, and became so finely honed that adherents of distinct positions on the subject were known as

Homoousions, Homoiousions, and Homoeans. A person holding the Old Testament view would find such notions ludicrous. However, the Greek language, rich in nouns, lends itself to finely-tuned distinctions, whereas Hebrew, which is rich in verbs, is eminently suited to practical description. The Greek verbal inheritance leads to the search for the touchstone of wisdom's riches in heady concepts rather than in day to day events.

To encounter God one only has to look around. In Romans 1:19, 20, Paul says, "All that may be known of God by men lies plain before their eyes; indeed God himself has disclosed it to them. His invisible attributes, that is to say his everlasting power and deity, have been visible, ever since the world began, to the eye of reason, in the things he has made." The undifferentiated One may be known in the spiral of creation: "Am I a god only near at hand, not far away? Can a man hide in any secret place and I not see him? Do I not fill heaven and earth? This is the very word of the Lord," (Jeremiah 23:23, 24).

The locus of the Christian faith is the presence of the creator in the person of Jesus of Nazareth. So total is this presence that to be one with Jesus is to be one with the Father. Although subsequent theological interpretation made the nature of attaining this union more complex, in the teaching of Jesus this union was attained by following his way of life. The writer of the fourth Gospel, reflecting the belief of the Church of that time, quotes Jesus as saying,

> Anyone who loves me will heed what I say; then my father will love him, and we will come to him and make our dwelling with him. (John 14:23)

The writer of Ephesians states specifically that this union exists and that we are called to attain full consciousness of that fact: "I kneel in prayer to the Father, from whom every family in heaven and on earth takes its name, that out of the treasure of his glory he may grant you strength and power through his Spirit in your inner being, that through faith Christ may dwell in your hearts in love. . . . So may you attain to the fullness of being, the fullness of God himself," (Ephesians 3:14–17, 19). The One whose being is our true being is further described in Ephesians as "one God and Father of all, who is over all and through all and in all," (Ephesians 4:6).

The union of creator and creation will be discussed further, for attaining awareness of this union is not only central to Christianity, but it is the purpose of the macrobiotic way of life. In *Natural Healing Through Macrobiotics,* Michio Kushi states, "The basic purpose of macrobiotic healing is to cure arrogance." He defines arrogance as what "occurs when we try to separate ourselves from nature and the universe." Separation of creator and creation is a powerful illusion, an unnatural state, a dis-ease which calls for a cure. The Christian knows this cure to be effected in the "inner being" through faith which manifests as love and denotes union with Christ. Macrobiotics sheds light on the path of the spiral of physical creation as it returns to the infinite One. There is no separation of living body and spirit, however, and the approaches of Christianity and macrobiotics speak of one, unified being—body, mind, and spirit interacting in an interdependent, ever-changing dynamic. The One "toward whom we move" is both the mover and the moved. That which writes in me reads in you.

The person who lived this truth, whose teaching and way of life is promised to grant us the realization that we and the Father are one, was sustained by a simple diet of grains, legumes, fresh vegetables, and fruits in season. This uncomplicated and unrefined fare, faith, and lifestyle produced events so profound that today we call them miracles.

Chapter 2

Everything Changes

"To everything there is a Season. . . ."
(Ecclesiastes 3: 1)

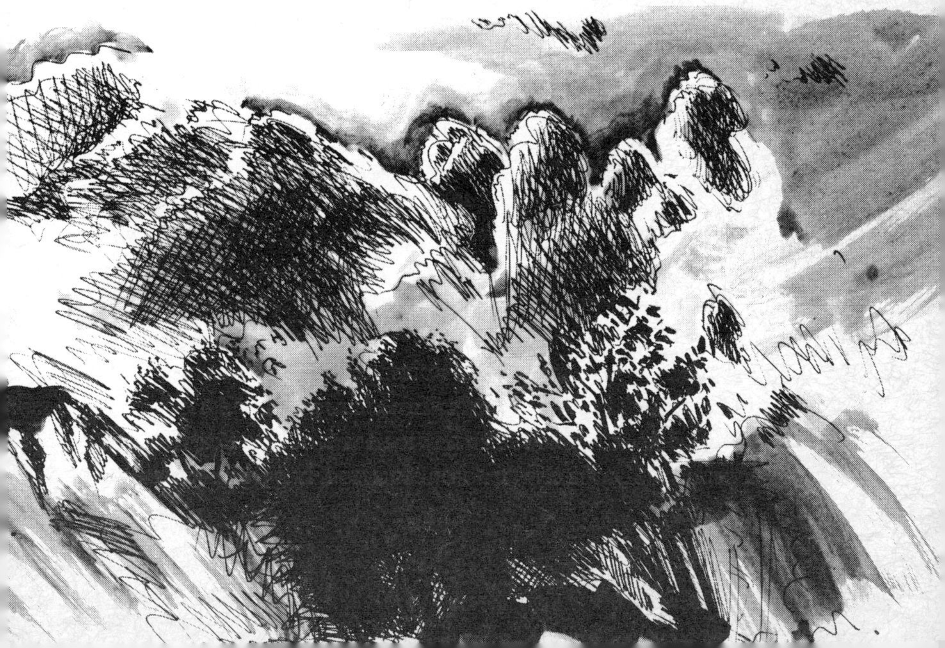

A MIDDLE EASTERN KING called the wise men of his court to him and said, "I want you to design a ring with an inscription upon it which will cheer me when I am sad and remind me that laughter, in time, is replaced with tears. Such an inscription will be easy to see and will keep me from becoming swept away by either elation or gloom." The court sages gathered to discuss their assignment and spent long days in debate. "It is true that happiness is fleeting, but then, too, even deep sadness eventually gives way to an equilibrium of emotions," they reasoned. At last they framed a statement small enough to fit the limited surface of a ring yet which incorporated the deepest truth of the inexorable law of change. The court jeweler produced the ring and it was presented to the king during a fitting ceremony. The inscription read, "THIS, TOO, SHALL PASS." The king was delighted, although one glance at the ring told him that there would be a time when his delight would end.

All things change. This fact may seem too simple to require any expounding upon, but, as ancient as perception of this truth may be, there seems to be something within the human condition which resists change. In macrobiotics this resistance is called inflexibility, in politics conservatism, in behavior stubbornness. The seven last words of any organization are: "we never did it that way before!" Is it the security of the familiar, fear of the future, or the threat of a loss of identity which gives rise to a maxim like, "The devil you know is better than the devil you do not know?" The possibility exists that the devil you do not know may not be a devil at all but a holy spirit. The devil you know is a devil, but what basic distrust of the universe produces the thought that the unknown is also devilish? Not all cultures share that view. Margaret Mead's work in Samoa, regardless of recent criticism, describes a people who were remarkably flexible as they made the adjustment from anthropologically primitive folkways to 20th Century civilization. There is nothing in the biblical tradition which supports fear of the future in and of itself, and the unknown is not automatically suspect.

Those of us raised in the West have been conditioned from

our earliest years to understand the universe as the product of basic, unchanging building blocks. We have been told that elementary blocks interact with other blocks in predictable ways to produce compounds of blocks the aggregate of which is the material world. When nuclear fission was controlled and made to split these blocks apart a chain reaction began which is still exploding a whole world view. This view is undergoing a meltdown as we move from what Fritjof Capra calls "the mechanistic view of life" to "the systems view of life." Capra's book, *The Turning Point,* describes the transition we are undergoing. The view of the mechanical universe described by Newton and elucidated by the philosophy of Descartes is giving way to an organic and ecological view. The mechanistic view has influenced medicine, psychology, and economics, and it is the basis of how we look at our world. During this century, modern physics has made discoveries which cannot be explained by the language and thought forms of the mechanistic view. A whole new view has arisen, ushered in by Einstein's revolutionary Special Theory of Relativity published in 1905. Subsequent interpretation and discovery has resulted in the fact that, for physicists, "the universe is no longer seen as a machine, made up of a multitude of separate objects, but appears as a harmonious indivisible whole, a network of dynamic relationships that include the human observer and his or her consciousness in an essential way."[1] Of particular interest here is that this new view is similar to that of saints and sages throughout recorded history.

When properties of the infinite One are ascribed to that which differentiates in an ever-changing dynamic from the One, then study of the differentiation becomes religion. As "the One" is forgotten, "this and that" become God. Newton believed that God created all that is, but he ascribed to the most basic building blocks a property formerly ascribed only to God: unchangeableness: "I am the Lord; I change not," (Malachi 3:6); "Long ago didst thou lay the foundations of the earth, and the heavens were thy handiwork. They shall pass away, but thou endurest . . . thou art the same and thy years shall have no end," (Psalm

102:25, 26, 27). The Epistle of James describes God as "The father of lights with whom there is no variation or shadow due to change," (James 1:17). The Judeo-Christian tradition holds that God does not change but that change is a characteristic of creation. After receiving a vision, Daniel declared, "Blessed be God's name from age to age, for all wisdom and power are his. He changes seasons and times," (Daniel 2:21).

The Book of Ecclesiastes, written toward the end of the Old Testament era and influenced by the Greek view that history is cyclical, poetically states the truth that everything changes:

> For everything its season, and for every activity under heaven its time: A time to be born and a time to die; a time to plant and a time to uproot; a time to kill and a time to heal; a time to pull down and a time to build up; a time to weep and a time to laugh; a time for mourning and a time for dancing; a time to scatter stones and a time to gather them; a time to embrace and a time to refrain from embracing; a time to seek and a time to lose; a time to keep and a time to throw away; a time to tear and a time to mend; a time for silence and a time for speech; a time for love and a time for hate; a time for war and a time for peace. (Ecclesiastes 3:1–8)

The idea that the One who creates the world of changing phenomena is, in essence, unchanging, has far-reaching implications for the practice of religion. Two areas where this unchangeableness seems to run counter to the practice and understanding of Christianity are those of prayer and revelation. What is expected by the faithful when petitionary prayer is addressed to God? God is unchanging. Is it expected that he will change his ways and manifest some condition or thing which does not now exist? The biblical God of history has set us in the midst of conditions and situations which are, literally, perfectly suited to what we need for our growth at the moment. Asking for a change in the situation is tantamount to telling God that he has made a mistake. This is a strikingly arrogant stance. Another interpretation of petitionary prayer must be in order. There are a pair of weather prayers in the 1928 Episcopal Book of Common Prayer, one for rain, one for fair weather, which demonstrate this point. The prayer for rain asks God to send rain, thus establishing that it is God who is believed to send rain. The prayer for fair weather asks that the "immoderate" rains cease, thus accusing God of being immoderate! These prayers are very old and reflect two things difficult for those outside the traditions of the Church to understand. We tend to project our present educational levels and scientific expertise back to those who lived in simpler and more naive times. The people who prayed those prayers were not interested in theological subtleties. They wanted their parched gardens drenched with life-sustaining water, or they wanted the threat of flood and destruction removed: "The God of history is at work here, let's pray to him to send rain or to stop it." The other factor which was at work in these delightful prayers is the familiarity which was understood to exist between the deity and humanity. God could be talked with and even given a talking to! Job did not hesitate to address God "in no uncertain terms": "Why didst thou bring me out of the womb? O that I had ended there and no eye had seen me, that I had been carried from the womb to the grave and were as though I had not been born. Is not my life short and fleeting? Let me be, that I may be happy for a moment . . . ," (Job 10: 18–20). If Adam walked with God in the cool of the evening in Eden, Job railed at his creator, and Jesus told his disciples to begin prayer with a word, Abba, best translated as, "Daddy," then surely letting God know that he had overdone the rain stands in a long tradition—familiarity with the One who is at the heart of our true self. This familiarity is in the true spirit of the Judeo-Christian tradition of so anthropomorphizing God that he becomes a "he" who can be believably portrayed by George Burns in the film *O God,* yet described by the writer of John as "love" and "light," or by Paul Tillich as "the ground of our being." I once had a parishioner of unshakable faith whose retarded son had been fathered by her former husband after their divorce. She had dedicated her life to work with the retarded and had total trust that God was working out his higher purpose come what may. One day during a counseling session she said, "Sometimes I think God has rocks in his head!" Anthropomorphism, creating God in our image, and the familiarity which permits a family argument with our father in heaven are threads woven through the fabric of the Christian faith.

The unchangeable One is asked to change not because he is expected to change but because creation always changes, and because a change will be effected in us by making the request: "Your Father knows what your needs are before you ask him," (Matthew 6:8). God does not have to be told what we need; *we* do. The petitionary prayer, then, is a prayer for the Spirit of God to pray with our spirit that our consciousness may be raised, that constructive thought forms may be built, that the positive side of what appears to be negative may be seen, that we may realize the whole of which we are an integral part. When a change is requested there must be an underlying understanding that, although the request is addressed to the infinite One who does not change, the change will be effected in this changing order as petitioned. This change will be as we desired in proportion to our faith. The intensity, without reservation, with which the prayer is prayed draws to us that condition requested: "If anyone says to this mountain, 'Be lifted from your place and hurled into the sea,' and has no inward doubts, but believes that what he says is happening, it will be done for him. I tell you, then, whatever you ask for in prayer, believe that you have received it and it will be yours . . . ," (Mark 11:22–24). A prayer for change is not a request for God to change his ways.

Since the undifferentiated One does not change, then what is the nature of revelation? The Bible is the history of what appears to be progressive revelation of God to humankind. This revealing can be described as occurring in two ways: by God's initiative and by the initiative of the seeker. The first way is the classic understanding of revelation, the latter more on the order of discovery. Christianity and Judaism both consider themselves "revealed religions" in that they claim to have arisen because God himself took the initiative of revelation rather than because the truth was discovered by the searching of believers. Daniel 2:47 describes God as a "revealer of secrets." Ecclesiasticus, in the Apocrypha, says that God "uncovers the traces of the world's mysteries." Although this revelation may come in the form of direct transmissions such as dreams, visions, angels, and other theophanies, the Biblical view is that the God of history reveals his nature in historical events. The eyes to see and the ears to hear, i.e., awareness (see Chapter 9) is all that is necessary on our part. This awareness comes through faith and through seeking and knocking as Jesus points out in Matthew 7:7. Those who were considered prophets in Old Testament times were those who were aware and could perceive God at work in everything that happened. "For the Lord God does nothing without giving to his servants, the prophets, knowledge of his plans," (Amos 3:7). In classical theology, to divide revelation into two distinct kinds is impossibly arbitrary. In the speech made in Athens, Paul says, "He created every race of men of one stock. . . . They were to seek God and, it might be, touch and find him; though, indeed, he is not far from each one of us, for in him we live and move, in him we exist," (Acts 17:26–27). The seeking and knocking is a created part of our nature and as much God at work as are apparent supernatural events.

The unchanging, undifferentiated One does not progressively reveal himself by his own initiative to a passively waiting creation. The One is found in the midst of the everchanging many which live and move and exist in him. A God which "speaks" through created events is not separate from that creation. The central figure of Christianity, Jesus of Nazareth, is the ultimate demonstration of the creator seen in creation. It is the belief of the Church that in Jesus' life the creator is seen, incarnate; that in this man the Holy Spirit, God at work in creation, is fully manifest. Peter's Pentecost speech captures this understanding and reflects the belief of the early Church when he says, "I speak of Jesus of Nazareth, a man singled out by God and made known to you through miracles, portents, and signs which God worked among you through him, as you well know," (Acts 2:22). This is not to say that in Jesus' life, death, and resurrection we find the only such revelation of the creator, or that those things which Jesus did are to be considered peculiar to him. His early followers performed what we consider miracles and the Church of the early second Century even believed that we would do greater things than Jesus had done (John 14:12). The statement, "The father and I are One," was never meant as an exclusive claim but a proclamation of the true relationship between the One and that which is a differentiation of the One.

God never changes. The power to work apparent miracles through faith never changes; "Jesus Christ is the same yesterday, today, and forever," (Hebrews 13:8). The same Spirit manifests in "diversities of gifts," (1 Corinthians 12:4). In the changing, created order we see the expression, the pressing outward, of the One creator whose unchanging law of manifestation is that everything changes. The Archbishop of Canterbury from 1942 to 1946, William Temple, said, "Unless all things are revelation, nothing can be revelation. Unless the rising of the sun reveals God, the rising of the Son of Man from the dead cannot reveal God." To separate God from his creation is like separating a ring from the gold of which it is made. Perhaps some elements within orthodox theology believe themselves able to make this separation, but a host of saints and sages as well as personal experience prove otherwise.

There is historic reason for the Church's rejection of pantheism, the belief that God and the universe are identical. Much of the reason bears on the Church's desire to steer a course clear of other religions in whose geographical area the gospel spread and whose tenets included such belief. However, the writings of believers like Dionysius, Erigens, Nicholas of Cusa, Meister Eckhart, and Jacob Boehme reflect subtle shadings of pantheism, and, in the words of Christopher Morley, "Men talk of 'finding God,' but no wonder it is difficult; he is hidden in that darkest hiding place, your heart. You, yourself, are part of him."[2]

The doctrine of the Trinity facilitates an understanding of how the unchanging One may be encountered in an ever-changing creation by elaborating the concept of the Spirit of God. God as spirit is not unique to Christianity. It has its roots in the oldest writings of the Old Testament and appears in the second verse of Genesis which describes the state of affairs at the beginning of creation: chaos, with God's Spirit *moving* over the face of the deep. The word which is translated "spirit" is, both in the Hebrew and the Greek, "a movement of air," "breeze," or "wind" and so "breath." Since breath is the prime indication that a body is alive, the association of spirit with the life principle is understandable. The prophet Zechariah says that God creates human spirit, (Zechariah 12:1) and Job says that God preserves it, (Job 10:12). The Spirit, then, belongs to God and is one with God. Paul develops this thought in Romans 8:9–17, and says in verses 14–16 that those moved by the Spirit of God are the sons of God and that, when we acknowledge this truth and cry, "Abba, Father" the Spirit of God joins with our spirit.

Spirit and wind are equated, too, in Jesus' explanation to Nichodemus in John 3:7, 8, "The wind blows where it wills; you hear the sound of it, but you do not know where it comes from, or where it is going. So with everyone who is born from spirit." In John 4:24, Jesus tells the Samaritan woman at the well that "God is Spirit." Wind and spirit appear as one at Pentecost when the disciples are gathered together and they hear a sound like the rushing of the wind, and the spirit alights on them as tongues of fire. The simile is an apt one as we try to put into familiar terms the nature of a fluid, dynamic, vivifying power eternally swirling into manifestation all that is.

This vivifying energy of the universe has been called by many names in both religion and science. Karl von Reichenbach referred to it as *Od*; Wilhelm Reich called it *Orgone;* (a most unfortunate choice in Victorian times); Russian scientists are calling it *bioplasmic energy;* in the Orient it is known as *Ki*, *Chi* or *Qi*. In India a whole science has evolved to work with this *prana,* an integral part of which is the conscious manipulation of the breath. Those who understand the practice of *pranayama* know that the connection of breath and spirit is more than just linguistic. In macrobiotics the life principle is described as manifesting through the interplay of two "forces," one whose direction comes from the earth and the other which descends from above. These forces are termed *Heaven's Force* and *Earth's Force*. To equate all of the above with the Holy Spirit is skating on theologically thin ice, but the universality of understanding is obvious since the belief in an ever-changing life principle is encountered, again and again, in widely divergent traditions.

Just as the wind feeds flames, is consumed by the fire and transmuted into a dynamic dance, so the wind of God's Spirit manifests as fire in many traditions. The breath which blew over the face of the deep in the creation myth of Genesis appears to Moses as a burning bush, leads the children of Israel as a pillar of fire through the wilderness, falls from the sky as fire on Mount Carmel at Elijah's bidding, alights as tongues of flame on the heads of those at the Pentoecost gathering, and speaks through John The Baptizer, who describes the advent of that same Spirit in the person of Jesus as a devouring fire.

The 5th Century B.C. Ephesian philosopher, Heraclitus, designated fire as the "primary substance" of the cosmos. He was derided by later philosophers who too literally interpreted his symbolic use of fire to describe the logos, the true law of all being. For Heraclitus this law was not a static and rigid form, but a dynamic principle of the harmony of opposites. When we consider the immense, fiery energy produced by atoms of hydrogen in a fusion reaction there may be more than symbolic meaning to Heraclitus' insight.

The universal law that everything changes is demonstrated in the dance of an open fire and in those same flames lies the power to transmute wood to gases and ash, oxygen to flame, and to transform the raw food appropriate to animals to the cooked food which marks the diet as human. The candles which grace the worship places of so many religions flicker with every movement of air as a reminder that there is within every element of creation a cosmic dance in progress, free and flowing like those born of the Spirit.

Faith in the naturalness and, therefore, the rightness of constant change anchors us to the unchanging, undifferentiated One and provides, in Bob Dylan's words, "a firm foundation when the winds of changes shift."[3] The purifying power in allowing the fire of change to consume the identity which has been constructed by interaction with the world, our persona, our mask, is described by Solomon, to whom the Book of Proverbs is traditionally attributed, "Can a man take fire in his bosom, and his clothes not be burned?" (Proverbs 6:27). St. Symeon, in the Philokalia, describes the process in more detail,

> And I say, can he who has in him divine fire of the Holy Spirit burning naked not be set on fire, not shine and glitter and not take on the radiance of the Deity in the degree of his purification and penetration by fire? For penetration by fire follows upon purification of the heart, and again purification of heart follows upon penetration by fire, that is, inasmuch as the heart is purified, so it receives divine grace, and again inasmuch as it receives grace so it is purified. When this is completed (that is, purification of heart and acquisition of grace have attained their fullness and perfection) through grace a man becomes wholly a god.[4]

Venite Spiritus, the hymn sung at ordinations, begins with the words, "Come Holy Ghost, our souls inspire and kindle with celestial fire." The divine spark within us is fanned into the consuming flame of union with the One. The Persian poet Farid al Din Atter tells the story of the moth and the candle:

> One night the moths gathered together, tormented by the desire to unite themselves with the candle flame. All of them said, "We must find one who can give us some news of that for which we seek so earnestly."
>
> One of the moths went to a castle far off and saw, within, the light of a candle. He came back and told the others what he had seen and began to describe the candle as intelligently

> as he was able to do. But the wise moth who was the chief of their assembly observed, "He has no real information to give us of the candle."
>
> Another moth visited the candle; he passed close to the light and drew near to it. With his wings he touched the flames of that which he desired; the heat of the candle drove him back and he was vanquished. He also returned and revealed something of the mystery, explaining a little of what union with the candle meant, but the wise moth said to him, "Your explanation is of no more real worth than that of your comrade."
>
> A third moth rose up, intoxicated with love, to hurl himself violently into the candle flame. He threw himself forward and stretched out his antennae toward the flame. As he entered completely into its embrace his members became red, like the flame itself. When the wise moth saw from afar that the flame had identified the moth with itself and had given to it its own light, he said, "This moth has accomplished his desire, but he, alone, comprehends that to which he has attained. No other knows it, and that is all."[5]

In Christian theology the beatific vision, or experience of union with the Divine Being, is the final destiny of the redeemed. This union is described as occurring in ecstatic states of consciousness where the believer is left bereft of perception of this world, as in the case of the Revelation of St. John The Divine, the last book in the New Testament. This union may also occur as an awareness of the overwhelming presence of God in daily affairs as described so simply by Brother Lawrence, the 17th Century Carmelite lay brother Nicolas Herman. Brother Lawrence's experiences and advice have been published in many forms under the title, *The Practice of the Presence of God,* and are an eminently practical guide to developing an awareness of the presence of the God of history in daily events. His work is discussed in detail in Chapter 12.

The New Testament demonstrates the centrality of belief in

this union in the faith of the early Church. The One (Mark 12:39) who is the Father of all (Matthew 23:10) is known by Jesus to be one with him (John 10:30) and, through "one faith" (Ephesians 4:5) in "one God and Father of all, who is over all and through all and in all," (Ephesians 4:6) the believer is made an "offspring of God in union with Christ Jesus," (Galatians 3:26). Throughout the writings of Paul and his school of theology this union with the One through union with the risen Jesus is a constant theme.

There is no recorded incident of Paul's having known Jesus of Nazareth before the crucifixion. Paul was a Pharisee, a home-based sect which stressed radical obedience to every aspect of the law. Their belief was that in this obedience one was assured of doing God's will. Pharisaism gained in power among the masses with the destruction of the temple in Jerusalem by the Romans in A.D. 70 and the subsequent loss of the Sadducees and temple authorities whose identity depended upon the existence of the building. Some scholars even claim that many of the confrontations which Jesus had with the Pharisees in the Gospels are an interpolation by those writing after the year 70 who were having problems with this group of "right wingers" and that the Pharisees were not as influential at the time of Jesus. Paul lived before the fall of the temple and he certainly gave the early followers of Jesus a difficult time. He presided over the death by stoning of Stephen, the first Christian martyr, and was on his way to Damascus to "arrest anyone he found, men or women, who followed the new way, and to bring them to Jerusalem," (Acts 9:2). His conversion is recorded in Acts 9:22, and 26, and is alluded to in 1 Corinthians 9:1; 15:8, and Galatians 1:15–16. He was knocked to the ground, blinded by a great light. He then heard the voice of Jesus who said, "Saul, Saul, why do you persecute me?" Paul had been persecuting the Church, the first followers, not the earthly individual Jesus of Nazareth. Yet, by the time the writer of Luke and Acts penned his words it was clearly understood that to persecute the Church was to persecute Jesus, himself. This point is an important one in discussing the union of believer with the Lord, because the use of Jesus' words in Acts 9:4 demonstrates one aspect of how this union was to be effected: through incorporation of the believer into the fellowship and life of the Church. Paul states this explicitly in Romans 12:4–5, "For just as in a single human body there are many limbs and organs, all with different functions, so all of us united with Christ form one body, serving individually as limbs and organs to one another." This same thought is re-phrased in 1 Corinthians 12:27, "Now you are Christ's body, and each of you a limb or organ of it." The rite initiating this incorporation into the body of Christ is that of Baptism (Romans 6:3) which Paul, himself, received from Ananias.

Paul also believed that each individual believer, initiated into the body of the Church, is one with Christ and even has the mind or, more accurately, the character of Christ, (1 Corinthians 2:16). It is the goal in the evolution of each person to "attain to fullness of being, the fullness of God himself," (Ephesians 3:19). For the churchgoer these words are familiar ones, and their revolutionary implications may not penetrate the anesthesia of familiarity. Paul does not see believers as separate from God, worshippers from afar, but destined to attain this unity ". . . measured by nothing less than the full stature of Christ," (Ephesians 4:14). Personal identity becomes lost with the realization that "the life I now live is not my life, but the life which Christ lives in me," (Galatians 2:20). Central to the teaching of this first theologian of the early Church is the theme of unity with the unchanging One whose wind-like spirit vivifies an ever-changing creation and is personified in the person of Jesus, now risen and, thus, accessible to all.

Everything which proceeds from the unchanging One changes, and, although continuity of consciousness may persuade us to the contrary, we, too, change from millisecond to millisecond. We are made new in this constant death and resurrection. The unity inherent in the changing order of the harmonizing of opposites should be a source of great hope. "This, too, shall pass," means that the situations perceived as difficulties are passing, the mountaintop experiences of elation cannot exist without the valleys of despair, and that to be obsessed with that which is ephemeral is to lose sight of the truth of our union with the eternal. The world's great religions teach that unity is our final destiny, and, if we can make our way through what Paul calls "a wilderness of words," (1 Timothy 1:6), we come to a place where all understandings are illuminated by the same light. On page 9 of *The Book of Macrobiotics,* Michio Kushi states:

> Everything in the universe is eternally changing, and this change proceeds according to the infinite order of the universe. This order of the universe was discovered, understood, and expressed at different times and in varying places throughout human history, forming the universal and common basis for all great religious, spiritual, philosophical, scientific, medical, and social traditions. The way to practice this universal and eternal order in daily life was taught by Fu-Hi, the Yellow Emperor, Lao Tzu, Confucius, Buddha, Nagarjuna, Moses, Jesus, and other great teachers in ancient times, and has been rediscovered, reapplied and taught repeatedly here and there over the past twenty centuries.

Because of our attachment to the *status quo* we often bemoan changes in our lives and consider them to be for the worse. We forget that change is the stuff of life. Grief, the normal human response to loss, may be overwhelming without the understanding that "this, too, shall pass." Each of us lives through major changes in life, the change called disease, the change called healing, the change called growing up, and each will experience the change called death. If our understanding matures we come to see that the changes are right, natural, even beneficial when viewed from the perspective of several months or years. It is also natural to feel overwhelmed in the stress of the moment of great change, but the law of change is our answer if we can, in the deepest part of our being, hold to the truth that the difficult moment will pass and that "God keeps faith, and he will not allow you to be tested above your powers, but when the test comes he will at the same time provide a way out, by enabling you to sustain it," (1 Corinthians 10:13).

The reading of those words comes far easier than the doing of them. To attain the inner and outer balance required to take everything in stride in full assurance that, come what may, all is right and natural, requires considerable attention to taking responsibility for our physical and spiritual wellbeing. It means taking responsibility for creating our reality, both for those things which seem to be drawn to us by chance and for the condition of the senses which perceive those things: "You must work out your own salvation in fear and trembling; for it is God who works in you, inspiring both the will and the deed, for his own chosen purpose," (Philippians 2: 12, 13). The macrobiotic way of life places great emphasis on personal responsibility for reality as we work out our own salvation. The dietary suggestions enable us to select and prepare food which will create a fit instrument for God to work in us, for us to work in God, regardless of the changes in climate and circumstance in which we may find ourselves. The practice of self-reflection according to our own preference and upbringing is an integral part of the practice of macrobiotics and the living of a fully human life. Appropriate physical exercise assures that the body is a suitable "temple of the Holy Spirit," (1 Corinthians 6: 19). Jesus of Nazareth and his disciples practiced such a life, eating locally grown grains, fruits and vegetables in season, praying together and meditating on the powerful events which were generated by their faith in the Father within and the imminence of his kingdom. They walked many miles and endured physical hardships in their travels. Through it all there was constant teaching, healing, forgiving, making whole that which seemed divided, and always the spirit of gratitude and celebration. One of the core, or authentic, sayings of Jesus is, "The Son of Man came eating and drinking . . . ," (Matthew 11: 19). This description of himself points to one of the most distinctive features of Jesus' way of life, was the cause of many disputes, (because of his choice of company with whom to eat and drink) and, ultimately, led to table fellowship as the normative worship experience of the Church from the last supper to this day in the stylized format of the Eucharist or Holy Communion.

The lifestyle practiced by Jesus was an integral part of the phenomenal flexibility which he demonstrated in the face of opposition. His teaching, "Resist not evil," and his willingness to shoulder his cross, albeit unjustly, should advise us to look very closely at stories about this man's life as we follow our dream in these rapidly changing and seemingly troubled times.

---

[1] F. Capra, *The Turning Point*, p. 47.

[2] Simcox, ed. *A Treasury of Quotations on Christian Themes*, p. 23.

[3] From the song, *Forever Young*.

[4] *Epiphany* (quarterly) Fall, 1982, p. 84.

[5] Ibid. p. 85.

Chapter 3

All Antagonisms are Complementary

"... Bless those who curse you. ..." (Luke 6:28)

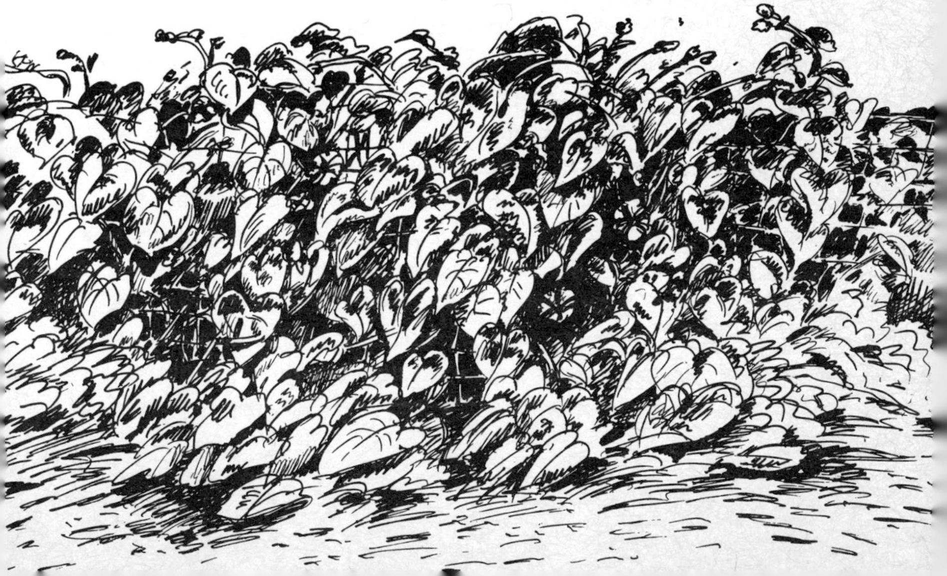

In one of Art Buchwald's most memorable columns, an official of The John Birch Society finds himself on an overseas flight sitting next to a Soviet agent. The agent is heading back to the Soviet Union to receive an award for the good work he has done in the United States. The John Birch official is to disembark in Europe to speak on the Communist threat in the United States. When they first discover each other's identity, conversation is cool. As the long flight progresses, they talk to pass the time and soon find that their successes are largely dependent upon each other. The Soviet agent has a sheaf of John Birch Society material to substantiate his claim that the Communists are, indeed, making inroads throughout the American scene. The John Birch official has an equally impressive collection of Communist Party propaganda to support his point of view. As they part, they wish each other well and acknowledge their need for each other in the jobs they are doing. It is a hilarious satire on the universal truth that all antagonisms are complementary; that, regardless of the strong position we hold on any issue, our position is vivified by the existence of an equally strong opposite position held by our antagonist.

The political right wing can only be identified as such because of the existence of radical politicians, and the political right is often identified by the name "reactionary," an identity gained by reacting to the opposition. Without light there would be no word for dark; men and women give each other sexual identity; we identify who we are to a great extent by who we are not. There could be no Protestant Christians without a theological point of view against which to protest.

The challenge of this principle is that it makes no value judgment upon the antagonisms involved but simply describes the truth of their complementarity. It is analogous to the nature of a teeter-totter or see-saw. The grammar school I attended had a solid set of these favorite playthings which were in use during every recess. We soon found out that to attempt to play on them without someone on the other end was something less than fulfilling. In fact, it was no play at all. A firm leg thrust could carry you into the air a little way, but the return to the ground was sudden and shocking. Once someone was on the other end, however, a whole new reality arose. Hardly any energy was required to soar to the limits of allowable movement, and the return trip was smooth and gentle.

The importance of the size of the opposite party was immediately apparent. Someone too heavy meant long moments teetering in the air before one's own end came back down, and that happened only at the behest of the partner. Even when a disparity in weight might cause problems, the situation could easily be overcome by the heavier person moving closer to you until the board would hold a relative balance when horizontal. I cannot remember thinking that the heavier or lighter person was better or worse for the weight differential. That was just the way it was, and, unless the difference was so great that the heavier person had to shinny so close to the middle of the board that the fun of flying was lost, a good time could be had by both partners.

Now I understand that, in that childhood game, we were acting out a universal principle including an implication which reaches far into the adult world: the person carrying the most weight must come closer to the position of the opposite party for there to be a "game" worthy of the name. Only a bully gloried in keeping his playmate dangling in the air because of their difference in weight. Even so, it happened quite often; it happens still.

The universe is a balancing act of infinite proportions, and our lives mirror in their microscopic way what is true of the macrocosm. Sometimes, when our psychological imbalance becomes extreme enough to be noticeable, we describe ourselves as having to work at just "keeping it together." Relationships, too, require that delicate touch when one partner becomes "the heavy" and the other partner has to accommodate in some way in order to keep any sense of balance. Understanding the principle of the complementarity of antagonisms is a key to the art of living. It is why some people are viewed as successes and others as people to avoid. The unforgettable teacher, the successful business person, the parents on the block that all the kids wanted to talk with—all understood the subtleties of this principle even if they might not be able to verbalize their understanding. Because of early training and sensitivity there are those for whom practical application of this principle just seems to come naturally.

There are indicators which point to understanding or lack of it. If difficulties are always understood as someone else's fault, creating a feeling of isolation as life passes by and an apparent pointlessness to activity, then this principle has eluded you. The key to its understanding is in taking the large view of any situation so that both your part and the contribution of the antagonism can be seen. This is, literally, the "macro" view. Details of this discussion appear in Chapter 11 on Awareness, but, suffice it to say, that as long as only one side of any situation is seen it is impossible to understand how that situation is given life by the opposing factors which create it. The result of the micro, or small, view is a feeling of helplessness in the face of mysterious and overwhelming odds. There is no human life which has not had the lesson of the complementarity of opposites presented to it over and over again. It is, after all, how reality manifests. Because we are so well trained by the Western bias to pick things apart rather than to put the parts together, this lesson goes unlearned for decades. Let us take a look at some classic instances of the working out of this principle.

Until the beginning of this century, physicists were certain that atoms were made up of tiny particles. These particles had names and electrical charges which kept them in balance, the positive charges equaling the negative charges in a complementary way. Experimental investigation in the early 1900's yielded some results which were totally unexpected. As the sophistication of experimental equipment developed, new aspects of atomic structure could be measured. Instead of the component parts of atoms appearing as particles, they appeared as waves! Not only did they appear as waves, but sometimes they appeared as particles depending, essentially, on how we looked at them. This means that these component parts can be considered as particles confined to a very small volume, and also as waves spread over a relatively large region of space. The puzzle of the dual nature of sub-atomic particles was solved by Niels Bohr who introduced the notion of complementarity. He considered the wave nature and the particle nature to be complementary descriptions of the same phenomenon, with each description being only partly correct in itself. Complementarity is now not only an established term in the field of physics, it is an essential part of the way physicists understand the natural order. Bohr even suggested that this concept might be useful outside the field of physics just as those who understand macrobiotic theory might suggest that the complementarity of opposites might be a useful notion within the field of physics! E. F. Schumacher, in his *Small is Beautiful,* a book which sounded a keynote for a whole generation, said, "The whole crux of economic life—and indeed life in general—is that it constantly requires the living reconciliation of opposites which, in strict logic, are irreconcilable."[1]

George Ohsawa offers a unique definition of faith which is biblically accurate and theologically irrefutable: "Understanding of how the Universe is truly constituted, the Unique Principle, the Kingdom of Heaven and its justice, the universal love that embraces all antagonisms so fully as to make them complementary —that is true faith, bringing infinite and eternal happiness to everyone."[2] By this definition Ohsawa points to the necessity of the believer's taking the largest view in seeing God at work in all that exists—a God of history, the divinity described in the Bible. The principle of complementarity, itself, becomes a description of what the Judeo-Christian tradition calls "God's love." This "love" is so vast that it even makes antagonisms complementary, working together in the divine economy, the plan for creation. This understanding is echoed in Paul, "All things work together for good to those who love God. . . ," (Romans 8:28). The important part of Paul's statement in this discussion is that all things "work together." It is a statement of complementarity.

As might be expected, the Bible is filled with stories of the complementarity of opposites which, in Schumacher's words, "in strict logic are irreconcilable." The creation of heaven and earth, the two aspects of the universe, is the creation of complementary opposites. From the interaction of various beings which populate these two realms arise many stories in both the Old and New Testament. We find manifestations of heaven and earth in opposition in legends of angelic visitations, in the appearance of Satan sent from the heavenly realm to accuse Job (the name Satan derives from the Hebrew root meaning "to oppose"), and in the "word of the Lord" spoken by the prophets, often to the dismay of the hearer and in opposition to the political establishment. This opposition is viewed by the biblical writers as examples of God working out his purpose and the ascendancy of God's ways over the intentions of those who are not able intuitively to fall in line with the divine economy, the natural order of the universe. There are times, as in Jacob's wrestling with the angel in Genesis 32, and in Job's loss of his home, family, and health, when the opposition seems overwhelming and the differences irreconcilable. Jacob's magnificent courage prevailed and won a blessing from the antagonist which entailed the change of Jacob's name to Israel—a name still very much in the news 3,500 years later. Job's lot has become synonymous with testing and faith in the face of terrible adversity. The Book of Job is one of the great statements of the difficulty of seeking the meaning of specific events and the futility of asking, "Why did this happen to me?" without considering the whole situation. Job clung to the degree of faith described by George Ohsawa and never lost his trust that, in Ohsawa's words, "the universal love that embraces all antagonisms so fully as to make them complementary" was at work in his phenomenal difficulties. Job's patience and problems certainly defied logical explanation.

There was no group of Old Testament personalities whose mission and image were more that of opposition than the prophets. The prophet was actually a professional person in ancient Israel. There were training schools for prophets, and the prophet was given license for behavior considered taboo by the rest of society, as in the case of Isaiah's going naked for three years

(Isaiah 20). When a prophet spoke he prefixed his remarks with, "Thus saith the Lord. . . ." Those listening knew that they were hearing God speaking. In the fierce monotheism of ancient Israel the prophet's ability to bring announcements from God gave him great power. The linguistic root of the word prophet has been lost, but in Hebrew the word seems to derive from the word "announce" and can mean either that the prophet makes or receives announcements from God. In the New Testament the Greek word means "to stand before." The prophet then becomes someone who stands before the king on behalf of the people, bringing their case to the sovereign and taking his pronouncements back to the people. Early prophets were a wild bunch, surrounded by miraculous happenings, able to predict the future (whether they were true or false prophets depended upon the accuracy of their predictions), free to scorn tradition, to practice confrontation politics, and say whatever they believed God said to them. John The Baptizer falls solidly within this tradition, and, like many before him, he was killed for what he said and for the threat which the freedom of his way of life represented. His head was served up on a silver platter.

The prophet Elijah, the greatest prophet of the Old Testament, was so revered that John The Baptizer was believed to be Elijah returned. Peter even reported, in Matthew 16, that some considered Jesus to be Elijah returned. A place at the table is set for Elijah to this day at the Jewish Seder at Passover time. Elijah's mission is one of antagonism and conflict out of which arises benefit for the people and religion of Israel. The identities of both Elijah and his antagonists are formed out of the conflict between them. It might be overstating the point to say that they needed each other, but their biblical importance is certainly dependent upon the complementarity of their opposition.

Following the reign of King Solomon, Israel was divided into two kingdoms, the northern kingdom called Israel and the southern kingdom, Judah. Ahab ruled the northern kingdom from 869 to 850 B.C. and is remembered to this day not so much as a political genius but as the husband of Jezebel. The story of his reign and the antagonism to that reign caused by Elijah can be found in The First and The Second Book of Kings (1:17–19, 21; 2:1–2). These books were penned sometime between 800 and 750 B.C. The interval between the events and when they were recorded allowed plenty of time for the embellishment of the dull, official records with legendary feats and stories of supernatural intervention. Ahab never saw Elijah's antagonisms as complementary. He considered Elijah to be the "troubler of Israel," (1 Kings 18:17).

The trouble arose over the introduction of the worship of a foreign God, Melkart, whose worship was imported by Ahab's foreign wife, Jezebel. A foreign wife was not a new event. Kings had contracted marriages for political convenience in Israel in the past, and the history of Europe often has been written around such arrangements. When Ahab married Jezebel, the daughter of Ethbaal, King of Sidon, he received considerably more than a positive effect on foreign policy. Jezebel was a woman of great influence in Ahab's realm. She came to Israel with four hundred prophets of Melkart and a religious devotion bordering on fanaticism. She saw to it that these prophets were supported at public expense, established a center of worship and even took her husband to "church" with her on occasion. In addition to the apparent commotion made by the presence of the overly zealous prophets, Ahab's predecessor, Jeroboam, had caused additional religious difficulty when he established a temple at Samaria to give the northern kingdom a center for its worship, as Jerusalem was for the southern kingdom. He had erected two gold-plated bulls as symbols of God's power and presence. Although bovines had been used in the religion of Israel in the past, with carvings of their horns on the altar and their blood used to seal covenants, the bull was a central symbol in the pagan religion of the area—the worship of Baal.

All of this may seem relatively insignificant from the perspective of 2,700 years, but, to the prophets of Yahweh, the God of the Jews, any move to introduce foreign theology and symbols was considered very serious, indeed. Any watering down of the faith which bound the Chosen People together could mean the eventual loss of identity, the failure of the covenant between God and Abraham, and the disappearance of the prime repository of monotheism. The success of Judaism's effort in this regard can be measured by the fact that in 1948, a state could be established and settled by a people who still had an ethnic/religious identity after 2,400 years without a homeland. The roots for that possibility lie buried in historical events such as these.

At some moment in the development of Jezebel's policies, Ahab found himself face to face with Elijah, God's champion. Elijah's communication with Ahab was brief and to the point: "I swear by the life of the Lord the God of Israel, whose servant I am, that there shall be neither dew not rain these coming years unless I give the word," (1 Kings 17:1). There is no report of Ahab's immediate response to this pronouncement, although the narrative later states that Ahab searched high and low for the prophet, who had immediately gone into hiding, for over two years. The drought came; famine spread throughout the land, and, in the third year, Elijah received word to return to Ahab.

Jezebel's religious fervor had resulted in the massacre of many prophets of the Lord, except for one hundred who had been hidden by Obadiah, Ahab's comptroller. Jezebel's effect on the religion of the people of Israel was significant enough that Elijah could accuse them of (understandably enough) "sitting on the fence" about their religion. Elijah's challenge was swift and sure: "Send and summon all Israel to meet me on Mount Carmel and the four hundred prophets of the goddess Asherah, who are Jezebel's pensioners."

The challenge involved sacrificing two bulls, one to each divinity, Baal and Yahweh. The bulls were prepared to be burned and the respective gods invoked. According to Elijah's challenges, fire must consume the sacrificed animals without being kindled by the prophets. Jezebel's prophets did their utmost, dancing wildly all morning and crying, "Baal, Baal, answer us." "But there was no sound, no answer" (1 Kings 18:26). Elijah mocked them, suggesting that perhaps they should call louder because their god might be in thought, or busy, or away, or asleep. They raved on through the afternoon, gashing themselves with knives and spears until they must have presented a bloody spectacle. Still there was no answer. Then Elijah repaired the altar which had been torn down, (apparently due to Jezebel's influence) had the offering doused with water several times just to make burning even more difficult, and he uttered a short invocation. Fire fell from heaven consuming everything including the water which had filled the trench around the sacrificial animal.

When the event was over, Elijah told Ahab to go home and eat and drink because the rain was coming. When Ahab told his wife what had happened she swore to kill Elijah within twenty-four hours. Elijah's reaction to this threat was interesting: "He was afraid and fled for his life," (1 Kings 19:3). He understood that Jezebel was the person of real power in the royal family.

Following the Mout Carmel event the people of Israel were turned from their "fence sitting" and again worshipped only the God of Abraham, Isaac, and Jacob. The demonstration of Elijah's power and the sovereignty of the God of Israel over any foreign deity was so convincing that the faith of the people was renewed. However, an additional event was required to convince Ahab, and this vineyard story demonstrates both Jezebel's cunning and Ahab's weakness. The story is found in Chapter 21 of The First Book of Kings.

Naboth owned a vineyard next to the palace. He had inherited it from his family and did not want to part with it. Ahab was so frustrated by the refusal of his purchase offer that he "Lay down on his bed, covered his face, and refused to eat," (1 Kings 21:4). It is easy to see how a person of even moderate inner strength could have had her way with Ahab. A person of Jezebel's power virtually could run the kingdom. She arranged for Naboth to be killed. Once this was accomplished she told Ahab to go and claim the vineyard because Naboth was dead. When he arrived at the vineyard Elijah was waiting for him. Ahab said, "Have you found me, my enemy?" Elijah answered, "I have found you because you sold yourself to do what is wrong in the eyes of the Lord." He then made a gory prediction that Jezebel would be eaten by dogs and all of Ahab's sons killed. Ahab had seen the Mount Carmel demonstration; this prophet's words were not to be taken lightly. He repented and was spared.

It is because of the power of Jezebel that Elijah is given occasion to manifest as one of the great luminaries of the Old Testament. It is Ahab's weakness compared with her power which gives Jezebel's influence the authority of royal permission. Without the religious fervor of the prophets of Asherah there could have been no confrontation on Mount Carmel and the returning of the people of Israel to the faith of their fathers. When his life was threatened by the powerful personality of Jezebel, Elijah understood the nature of his opponent well enough to be afraid and flee for his life. Although the massive demonstration on Mount Carmel was required to convince the whole populace, it was an event of a far more personal nature which brought Ahab to repentance: the killing of Naboth and the one-to-one meeting with Elijah.

The story of Elijah and Ahab is filled with examples of complementarity made potent by the extreme nature of the antagonism. Elijah's singlemindedness and unswerving faith is drawn to his king's doublemindedness and vacillation just as surely as the north pole of one magnet is drawn to the south pole of another. That same attraction brings Elijah to Carmel to face the feckless prophets of Baal. The equivalent personal power of Elijah and Jezebel drives him into hiding when he is threatened with death and keeps them physically apart throughout the story. Out of the antagonisms comes a working together for good; the orthodoxy of the religion of the northern kingdom and the whole history of the Jewish people is affected by the events which unfold in this story.

It is another prophet, Amos, who announces that God works as actively in the opposition as in the lives of those who consider themselves to be his Chosen People. In the development of the theology of the Old Testament, Amos' prophecies stand as a watershed. Although it was understood that God was at work in the personalities and events of the people of Israel, as in the confrontations between Elijah and Ahab, it was thought that the surrounding enemy countries were simply kingdoms which represented a threat to the existence of Israel and were totally outside the domain of the God of Israel. The scope of God's influence, interest, and plan is expanded in the theology introduced by the shepherd and "pincher of Sycamore fruit," Amos, from the period around 750 B.C. His message describes a God who is as interested in the shortcomings of the people of the surrounding enemy nations as he is in the sins of the people of Israel.

The Book of Amos begins with a stylized, almost song-like series of prophecies about the cities whose inhabitants were so hated by the Israelites—Damascus, Gaza, Tyre, Edom, Rabbah. Each stanza begins with the words, "For crime after crime of. . . ." It is easy to picture the people gathered around the prophet on his "soap box" in the city square denouncing these criminal enemies amid cheers as each city is described receiving its punishment at God's hand. Then, in the fourth verse of the second chapter, Amos begins a new stanza, "These are the words of the Lord: For crime after crime. . . ." The people strained to hear which enemy was to be punished next, and then came the shock: "of Judah I will grant them no reprieve. . . ." Judah was the southern kingdom of the divided nation; God was going to punish his own people with a passion equal to the way he dealt with the enemy! Amos is speaking to the people of the northern kingdom and his listeners may well have felt that those people to the south with their own king, their center of worship in Jerusalem, and somewhat different ways probably were deserving of God's wrath, too. Then Amos begins a new stanza with the now familiar opening words, "for crime after crime . . . of *Israel*. . . ." Those gathered to hear the prophet were stunned and must have thought, "But that's *us*! You mean God will punish *us* just as he deals with our enemies?"

In Amos' words we see the beginnings of the understanding that the whole history of the world "works together." Even the specific punishment levied upon these people comes because of their own doing, as a balance to their willing flaunting of the law of the Lord, the order of the universe: ". . . because they have spurned the law of the Lord and have not observed his decrees, and have been led astray by the false gods . . . Therefore . . ." (Amos 2:4). The result of this lawlessness is perfectly natural; it is logical; it is as extreme as the behavior of which it is the result. The behavior, to be specific, is: ". . . they sell the innocent for silver, and the destitute for a pair of shoes. They grind the heads of the poor into the earth and thrust the humble out of their way. Father and son resort to the same girl, to the profanation of my holy name. Men lie down beside every altar on garments seized in pledge, and in the house of their God they drink liquor got by way of fines," (Amos 2:6–8). This is a clear description of the truth that we reap what we sow. It is a declaration that the universe tends toward balance regardless of the religious or political persuasion of those being dealt with. The powers of heaven may seem to be in opposition to those of earth, but, in the total view, those powers work together to create the whole.

In all the Bible there is no figure surrounded by greater antagonism than Jesus of Nazareth. The whole recorded Christ event, from the moment of his conception to the post-resurrection experiences of the early Church, is filled with apparent difficulty, opposition, and breakdown in communication. The gospel accounts of Jesus' ministry read like a catalogue of confrontations. Jesus' earthly life is ended with phenomenal pain and anguish for him and his followers as they watch him nailed to a timber and hanged to dehydrate under a searing sun. The events which follow the crucifixion and which are supposed to be filled with joy in fact recount the beginning of three hundred years of persecution. Followers were subjected to torture, death by stoning, crucifixion, being thrown to lions, and massacred by the government and religious authorities. Today the stories of the beginning of these vicissitudes are called the gospels, the "good news." They can only be called "good" by an interpreter who understands that there is a "universal love which embraces all antagonisms so fully as to make them complementary." Ohsawa's definition of faith applies here with all the force he intended it to carry. The early Christians went to their deaths singing! Their master went to his death forgiving those who were at that moment driving nails into his wrists.

Without considering the extremely delicate and complex question of historicity, let us consider some of the events in the life of Jesus as recorded in the gospels from the oral tradition of the early Church.

The opposition and seeming difficulty begins before Jesus is even born, at the moment of his conception. A "young girl" (the Hebrew word for "virgin," since to be a young girl in that society was to be a virgin) is confronted by the archangel Gabriel and told that she is to be pregnant. She is engaged to be married but, as rigid custom dictates, has not had sexual intercourse with her espoused nor with anyone else. In the world of her day, this announcement of pregnancy was like a death sentence. Her beloved, of course could not be expected to marry a woman expecting someone else's child, and her future as a prostitute is assured. Mary must have realized all this in the moment of the announcement. Her alarm must have been ameliorated somewhat by the presence of the radiant, angelic messenger and the words of assurance she received. It is also possible that her fright at being so confronted left her barely able to comprehend the message. Her reaction is swift, however, and once she finds out that what she considered impossible is not only possible but the fact of the matter she says, "I am the Lord's servant; as you have spoken so be it," (Luke 1:38). Her response is one of great faith. God is at work; God is good; what is happening now is good. An event which runs opposite to all her expectations is received with grace and with faith in its rightness.

Joseph, too, is visited by an angel in the gospel stories. He is told what would be considered by his society to be the bad news—that he must fly in the face of social custom and contract the marriage. He immediately got out of bed and "took Mary home to be his wife . . ." (Matthew 1:24). As with Mary, Joseph acted swiftly and gracefully without quarrel.

The striking characteristic in this and the other confrontation stories is the attitude of the people confronted. Those of faith obey with dispatch as if to say, "Regardless of how many problems this raises for me, the hand of the divine is at work here, and that same hand will lead me to realization of ultimate rightness." Such an attitude is an explicit indication of good health, both spiritual and physical. In George Ohsawa's six conditions of health the sixth condition is precision in thought and action. Ohsawa states that a person "who enjoys good health is able to make sound judgments swiftly and instinctively, acting with speed and precision. . . . Those who are prompt, quick and precise are always prepared to meet any challenge, any emergency, any accident. They enjoy good health."[3] Michio Kushi reflects this thought:

> Whenever there is no difficulty there is no development. If we avoid such difficulties, we eventually become weaker and decline after momentary comfort. Let us welcome, at any time, any sort of difficulties. Let us appreciate them as our teachers.[4]

The popular statement of this truth is: "No pain, no gain," and, to the Christian, "No cross, no crown." These are all statements of the complementarity of opposites.

The story of Jesus continues with the difficult trip to Bethlehem at the time of his birth (Luke 2:1–7) and the flight to Egypt necessitated by Herod's threat to kill all children in the Bethlehem area (Matthew 2:16). Jesus' parents are upset at his desire to ask questions of the doctors of the law when he was expected to be on the return trip to Nazareth after the trek to Jerusalem for the Passover celebration (Luke 2:41–52). There is no indication that the holy family complained at having to make the trip to Bethlehem, at being turned away at the inn to have their baby in a place built for animals. They go to Egypt obediently, trusting that it must be best and forever leaving their mark on the Coptic Church of North Africa which to this day has special veneration for the holy family. At the time announced, they return to Nazareth, where Joseph resumes his trade of carpentry. When they confront their twelve-year-old son about his absence on the journey home from the Passover celebration he simply tells them his reason, and that is sufficient for them.

Later, Jesus asks John The Baptizer to administer the symbolic ablution of baptism and is confronted by John's unwillingness to do so. The forty days and nights in the wilderness following the baptism culminate in the story of Jesus' being confronted by the devil and tempted to use divine powers to effect material gain and fame (Matthew 4: 1–11). Following what must have been a few, short weeks of public ministry Jesus comes to his home town and attends worship in the local synagogue. Here he reads the Isaiah passage:

> The Spirit of the Lord is upon me because he has anointed me; he has sent me to announce good news to the poor, to proclaim release for prisoners and recovering of sight for the blind; to let the broken victims go free, to proclaim the year of the Lord's favor. (Luke 4: 18, 19)

Following the reading, Jesus spoke a few brief words which had a devastating effect upon the attitude of his home town friends toward him: "Today, in your very hearing this text has come true." In Luke 4, verses 28 and 29 we read the result, "At these words the whole congregation was infuriated. They leapt up, threw him out of town, and took him to the brow of the hill on which it was built meaning to hurl him over the edge."

Jesus' dream is God's plan and his ministry is one of living that dream as a demonstration of its possibility—the dream and the possibility of unconditional love and trust between created and creator, between all children of the same father. He follows this dream with a resolution born of certainty. There is no vacillation in his course, no tempting him from the path with promises of material gain, not even an indication that rejection by his former neighbors caused a moment of hesitation. When he was taken "to the brow of the hill," he must have realized that, indeed, this was not going to be easy. His reaction at that moment is indicative of his resolution and the power of such one pointed resolve: "But he walked straight through them all and went away," (Luke 4:30). Their opposition is galvanized by the sure resolve with which he announced, "Today, in your very hearing this text has come true." His certainty is vivified and reinforced by their fury. He walks "straight through them all." Later in his teaching, he describes the necessity for such radical obedience to one's understanding and intuition when he says, "Straight is the gate and narrow is the way that leads to life . . ." (Matthew 7:14).

Opposition to Jesus' mission and message came from several identifiable groups. First, there was opposition from the people at large, the hearers of the word who gathered around him or encountered him in the marketplace. Second, the religious authorities became increasingly concerned as his fame spread. Both the Sadducees, who were the priestly class associated with temple worship in Jerusalem, and the Pharisees—the strict constructionist, law-based, conservative party among the people—sought to trip him up, to test him, and even to put him to death early in his public ministry. A third, and unexpected, opposition came from his own disciples who are portrayed as disagreeing with him, squabbling among themselves, and refusing to hear what he said. At the end of the public ministry there is a fourth and expected quarter of opposition by the Roman authorities who saw possible political consequences in the gathering of thousands around this itinerant preacher and in the proclamation that he was "King of the Jews."

Jesus deals with opposition from the people by "walking straight through them" both literally and figuratively as he exercises his ministry of love and forgiveness. Soon their opposition wanes as the overwhelmingly convincing nature of the healings which surround him outweigh the blasphemy of those who consider him to be the "Son of the living God," (Matthew 16 : 16). This opposition is rekindled momentarily by rabble rousers at the trial before Pilate, but the confrontations between Jesus and the Pharisees, Sadducees, and disciples give occasion for much of his teaching. He is virtually silent before the governmental authorities. What are his teachings on antagonism and what attitude underlies them?

Jesus was well schooled in the Hebrew scriptures. He knew them well, quoted them often, and he held the biblical faith in the omnipotence of God. He knew, as had the biblical writers, that God is good and that his creation is good. He understood that the love of God encompasses both sides of any situation, that heaven and earth are not two but one. The Jewish-Christian writer of the Gospel of Matthew reports Jesus as saying that he had come only to "the lost sheep of the house of Israel," (Matthew 15: 24) but John's Gospel, written for gentile Christians, reports Jesus as offering salvation to a Samaritan woman. He heals the daughter of the Canaanite woman, casts out demons from the Gerasene demoniac, and heals the son of the Roman Centurion. There is no limit to the Spirit of God who, like the wind, "blows where it wills," (John 3: 8). He may well have seen the scripture written between the time of the Old Testament writings and the New Testament known as Ecclesiasticus.[5] In Chapter 42, verses 24, 25, the writer states, "All things go in pairs, one the opposite of the other; he has made nothing incomplete. One thing supplements the virtues of another. Who could ever contemplate his glory enough?"[6] This quotation states the universal principle that all antagonisms are complementary perhaps more succinctly than anywhere else in the Bible. This principle obviously was known in the near East at the time of Jesus even more explicitly than just by inference of its understanding in Old Testament writings.

Jesus' teaching is also explicit in revealing his understanding of complementarity. The disciples saw in their master the promise of the return to glory of the kingdom of Israel. Their notion of the nature of the Messiah was based on scriptural prophecy. He was to be of the lineage of David; he was to be a military as well as religious leader; he was to usher in a whole new political and spiritual realm with Jerusalem at its center. The prophet Zechariah even described the events which would herald the coming of this new age and the restoration of the fortunes of Israel with its resumption of primacy among the nations of the world. Chapters 12–14 of Zechariah describe these events on the day when the anointed one, the King, the Messiah, the Christ[7] would bring about restoration of the kingdom and the reign on God on earth. Because their expectations were so well established, they could not comprehend a statement like, "My kingdom is not of this world," (John 18: 36). They were not only expecting that his kingdom would be very much of this world but that they would each have an important place in its governance. This expectation is reflected in the request for assurance by James' and John's mother that her two sons be installed in powerful positions: "I want you," she said, "to give orders that in your kingdom my two sons here may sit next to you, one at your right and the other at your left," (Matthew 20: 22). Jesus responds with, "You do not know what you are asking," (Matthew 20: 22). There is no place in her expectations for the Messiah to encounter difficulty. As God's anointed, he would simply sweep aside any possible difficulty and assume the restored throne of King David. These are expectations which fail to take into account the necessity of opposites and the galvanizing effect which difficulty creates.

Against this background, the story of Peter's confession that he believes Jesus to be the Messiah is an apt demonstration of Jesus' understanding, and Peter's ignorance, of the law of complementarity. Jesus and his disciples set out for the villages of a region known as Caesarea Philippi. On the way Jesus asks them, "Who do men say that I am?" (Mark 8: 27). They give him a variety of answers, some enigmatic, as in "John The Baptist," reported by Matthew, Mark, and Luke; Matthew also reports, "Jeremiah . . ." (16: 14), all three evangelists report "Elijah . . ." and "one of the prophets." After hearing that the people think he is the reincarnation of these famous personalities,

Jesus asks, "But who do *you* say that I am?" (Matthew 16:15, Mark 8:29, Luke 9:20). Peter is the only one to answer and says, "You are the Messiah." Immediately Jesus "began to teach them that the Son of Man has to undergo great sufferings, and to be rejected by the elders, chief priests, and doctors of the law; to be put to death, and to rise again three days afterward. He spoke about it plainly," (Mark 8:31, 32). There could be no messianic victory, no glory, without its opposite—suffering and rejection.

> Peter took him by the arm and began to rebuke him. But Jesus turned around, and, looking at his disciples, rebuked Peter. "Away with you, Satan," he said, "you think as men think, not as God thinks." (Mark 8:32, 33)

Jesus' frustration at their lack of understanding surfaces; they have a lot to learn. Jesus even considers ignorance of this truth satanic!

The Sermon on the Mount, a collection of sayings attributed to Jesus, reads like a manual of instruction on universal principles. The fifth chapter of the Gospel of Matthew records these teachings, which include accepting insult and persecution gladly, (5:12) recognizing persecution as a blessing, (5:10) and loving enemies, (5:44). This latter teaching runs contrary to the wisdom of the world and is of particular interest to the discussion of complementarity. The full statement is, "Love your enemies, bless those who persecute you, do good to those who hate you, pray for your persecutors and those who treat you spitefully; only so can you be children of your heavenly Father who makes his sun rise on good and bad alike, and sends rain on the honest and the dishonest," (5:44–46). Verse 48 gives an admonition and an explanation, "You must, therefore, be all goodness just as your heavenly Father is all good." Jesus knows that he is one with the Father and that, "A pupil is not superior to his teacher; but everyone, when his training is complete, will reach his teacher's level," (Luke 6:40). He expects all his disciples to attain his consciousness of unity. God-consciousness sees beyond all antagonisms to the complementarity they encompass.

We are to love our enemies and bless those who curse us because, in the words of the Jesuit, John Powell, "We are created by those who love us and those who refuse to love us." Love of, and respect for, self is presupposed in this understanding. If we hate who we are, we must hate those who created us through our interactions with them. Jesus' summary of the law, "love your neighbor as yourself," (Matthew 22:39) makes this presupposition as well. So deep has become the phenomenon of dissatisfaction and dislike for who we are that whole movements in psychology have arisen to counteract the tendency. The Transactional Analysis school whose battle cry is, "I'm O.K., you're O.K." is such an organization. Paul says, "By God's grace I am what I am," (1 Corinthians 15:10). But our interaction with those who love us and those who are afraid to love us is not a capricious thing. We are led to each person and situation as an ongoing part of the act of creation. We are drawn to each other through the working out of the principle that we reap what we sow. Each moment, more especially the times of interpersonal interaction, are occasions of creation, times of blessing, times for gratitude—even when they appear to be times of persecution and suffering. This teaching is far, indeed, from the "wisdom" of the world. There is consolation in knowing that "the wisdom of this world is foolishness to God," (1 Corinthians 3:19). The world sees "in part" and the consciousness which is one with the Father sees the whole. The sun rises on us all; the rain falls upon us all. That which today seems terrible is recognized as a blessing from the perspective brought by time.

There is a day in the Christian calendar which most vividly demonstrates not only the complementary nature of antagonisms but the necessity of opposites in the manifestation of the whole: the day Jesus was crucified. Those who had followed him during his short ministry and who harbored their mad dream of his political leadership watched in horror as they saw their master die a criminal's death. All the promise of their days together was gone. It was over. Accounts of this and following days report that some simply went back to doing what they had done before he called them away from their nets to become "fishers of men." There was no question now of who would sit next to whom in his kingdom. The flame of hope and expectation had been snuffed out on a hillock outside the city of David, named for the king whose heir Jesus was, whose glorious monarchy was to be restored. There could not have been a blacker day for that band of followers. Jesus, had "set his face resolutely towards Jerusalem" (Luke 9: 51) when he understood what lay ahead for him. His followers had "rebuked him," refused to hear his description of what would happen even when "he spoke about it plainly," (Mark 8: 32) and reacted to the events surrounding the crucifixion with desertion, denial, and doubt. They must have been in a state of phenomenal confusion and loneliness on that Saturday between Friday and the first Easter.

The reports which began coming in about the tomb being empty and encounters with a risen Jesus were met with skepticism, to say the least. His followers seemed totally unprepared for the resurrection events. They had seen the dead rise in Jesus' healings; he had told them specifically what the sequence would be from crucifixion to resurrection, and, most importantly, he had lived a demonstration of the life of joy which comes with the realization of the unity of creation and creator. Still, they were not ready.

Our expectations weave the fabric of the filter through which our world flows. Limited expectations leave us able to see only limited possibilities. Jesus lived a life of tremendous spiritual abundance. The pictures painted by the gospel accounts show him to be open to whatever happened, trusting in its intrinsic worth, ready to accept even crucifixion as a necessary part of a far greater whole.

Once the resurrection encounters were so widespread that even the original "doubting Thomas" could no longer deny their reality, a new spirit filled the followers of Jesus. Timid lives became bold, doubts turned to certainty, persecution and death were faced with song, ancient traditions were discarded. A new day had dawned which was as bright as that Friday of death had been dark. Life and death had been demonstrated to be parts of one whole, an eternal interplay of heaven and earth. The vertical and the horizontal had come together in the cross; "the hopes and fears of all the years" had met in this one known by his followers as Son of God and Son of man. The worst day in their lives now could be called Good Friday.

All antagonisms are complementary; bless those who curse you.

---

[1] Schumacher, *Snall is Beautiful,* p. 258.

[2] Ohsawa, George, *You are All Sanpaku,* p. 85.

[3] Ibid. pp. 63–64.

[4] Kushi, *The Book of Macrobiotics,* p. 97.

[5] This book represents the wisdom of the time and follows closely the teaching of the Torah, the Jewish scriptures. It is now part of the Apocrypha, a collection of writings from the intertestamental period recognized by some denominations of Christendom.

[6] The word "virtue" here refers not to some trait of ethical excellence but to inherent power or potency, as in the healing of the woman who touched the hem of Jesus' garment and "Jesus, immediately knowing in himself that virtue had gone out of him, turned him about in the press. . . ." (Mark 5:30)

[7] All these words share a common meaning due to the act of anointing the king with oil, or, in Greek, "Chrism," as the outward sign of coronation.

Chapter 4

There are No Two Things Identical

"Many, O Lord, my God, are thy wonderful works . . . if I would declare and speak of them, they are more than can be numbered." (Psalm 40: 5)

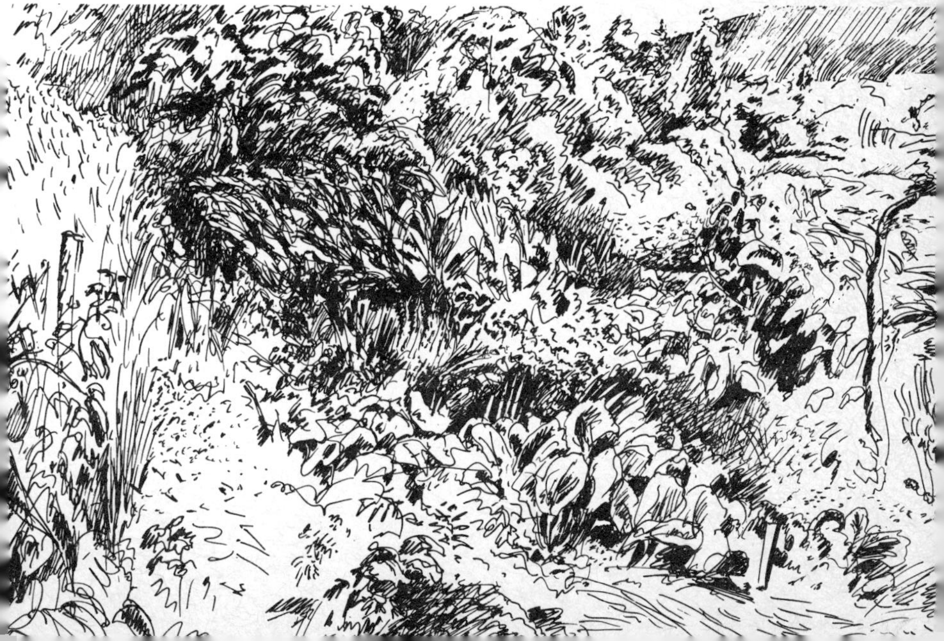

HUMANKIND HAS ALWAYS HAD A FASCINATION with the phenomenal variety within creation. From the earliest times there have been hymns of praise for the number of stars. Today there is so much interfering light that most of us have had little chance to see the true abundance of stars. To the desert-dwelling semitic people, every clear night brought a glorious spectacle. The Old Testament uses the number of stars to show God's creativity and omniscience: ". . . he who numbers the stars and names them one and all," (Psalm 147 : 4). Abram, later to become Abraham, is promised, "Look up into the sky, and count the stars if you can. So many, he said, shall your descendants be," (Genesis 15 : 5). The assumption is that one could not even begin to count the vast number of stars. In actuality there are about 2,500 stars visible to the unaided eye on a clear night. Still, they dominate the sky and, in their very being, praise their creator: "Praise him sun and moon; praise him all you shining stars," (Psalm 148 : 3). They stand as a supreme example of the variety within creation, both in their sheer numbers and their individuality, some twinkling, some bright, some faint. A trip to the deserts of the Southwestern United States several years ago convinced me of the dominance of the reality of stars to the desert dwelling people who slept under them. Astronomers now tell us that their true number is in the trillions.

Another phenomenon in great abundance is sand, and sand is used extensively as a simile for uncountable numbers. In many places in the Old Testament the number of the children of Israel is likened to the number of grains of sand, if not in actuality at least in promise. "How deep I find thy thoughts, O God, how inexhaustible their themes! Can I count them? They outnumber the grains of sand; to finish their count, my years must equal thine," (Psalm 139 : 18). Here is introduced another uncountable aspect of the creator and creation—the "thoughts" of God, the physical and spiritual principles and laws in accordance with which creation operates.

Different people have referred to this variety within creation in different ways. In the religion of the Sikhs of Northern India, the principle of no two things being identical is referred to as "eight million things." In Buddhism, it is "ten thousand things." In Judaism and Christianity it is, "Everything that he hath made." James Herriot, the Yorkshire veterinarian, has had huge success with his series of anecdotal books titled after lines of the Christian hymn, "All Things Bright and Beautiful." The titles of his books follow the lines of the hymn's first stanza, "All things bright and beautiful/All creatures great and small/All things wise and wonderful/The Lord God made them all." This children's hymn not only makes note of the variety of created things but, more importantly for this discussion, that this variety contains within it a sacred quality as parts of a whole creation sprung from and participating in divine energy. The psalmist sums it up in the fifth verse of Psalm 40: "Great things thou hast done, O Lord my God; thy wonderful purposes are all for our good; none can compare with thee; I would proclaim them and speak of them but they are more than I can tell."

In a recently translated, comparatively dispassionate explanation of this universal principle published in the Spring 1984, edition of the magazine, *Macromuse,* George Ohsawa is quoted:

> The principle of non-duplication arises because everything keeps moving towards its opposite: mountains, rivers and rocks, nations, the earth, the planets and suns never stop for one instant. They all are floating, flying, ephemeral, all in movement. Mountains are waves which rise and descend, then disappear into nothingness. All changes, including equilibrium, are produced by opposite crossing motions projected onto the screen of absolute infinity.[1]

A moment of reflection will reveal why this principle is true, although we may, at first, insist that molecules must be identical. How about identical twins? But no two molecules can occupy the same space at the same time. They must be in different places. The very fact that identical twins are born one after the other makes them different from the moment of birth. Experientially they are anything but identical. With the seal of validation which the Nobel Prize brings, we now recognize the phenomenon of "jumping genes." Even genetic similarity may not be true for "identical" twins.

Ohsawa's explanation reminds us, again, that, in the macrobiotic view, recognition of the principle of universal change prevents us from holding things in a static state even for the purpose of examination. In his words, "They are all floating, flying, ephemeral, all in movement." How different this is from Western science's attempt to fly in the face of reality, establish a condition of standard temperature and pressure, and pick apart creation as if it could be stopped and examined. The closest we have come to "stopping" creation is in the field of nuclear physics where phenomena are measured in such tiny time fractions that they are almost "frozen." When this is done, however, creation falls into an absurd disarray, manifesting sometimes as particles, sometimes as waves, sometimes there, sometimes not, blinking on and off with equal time spent in being and non-being. The implications of a world which half the time does not exist are as many as "the stars in the sky!" In the large, or macro, view, there is no isolating the parts from the whole. The strand can only be understood in terms of its relation to the everchanging web. The description of a creation in constant movement is reminiscent of the Genesis creation story which describes God's spirit as "moving over the face of the deep," and Jesus' explanation to Nicodemus that the Spirit is like the wind, producing movement although invisible. Jesus says that those who are born of the Spirit also exhibit this unpredictability and freedom.

This principle of non-duplication should come as welcomed news to those who consider themselves just one more cog in the wheel of life. In an era which has produced so much standardization, it is difficult not to see one's self as standardized as well. Take heart! Creation does not work on the production line principle. There are no two things identical, especially human beings. Each of us is unique and that uniqueness implies that each individual is of great value and absolutely necessary in making up the whole created order. When a product is produced in a "limited edition" it becomes of greater value as a collector's item over the years. Human beings, like the rest of creation, are made in extremely limited editions— one each. Therefore, what each of us has to offer as our part of the whole cannot be offered by anyone else. Not only is each contribution as unique as the contributor, but even a lack of contribution is unique. No two people can waste time in exactly the same way in exactly the same place with exactly the same thought processes.

From the moment of conception when no one else is conceived at that moment in that mother's body, to the profound effect which each unique prenatal diet has on development, to the fact that no other baby is born to that mother at that moment, each person is born into this world with millions of unique qualities. When uniqueness at birth is overlayed with years of "one of a kind" relationships, geographical location, and dietary peculiarities and experiences, the principle of non-duplication as applied to human beings becomes obvious. Not only is each person unique physically and psychologically, but each of us treads a unique spiritual path. We are confronted with our own lessons to be learned, blocks to that unpredictable and free life of the Spirit to be removed, issues of interpersonal relationships to be resolved. These issues plumb the depths of human nature and, by the challenge of their variety, call into being our own peculiar strengths and weaknesses.

We gain our identity through interacting with our world and know ourselves, in part, through the image of our internal knowledge and how that image squares with the way our lives are lived out in the world. Only each of us can know our own inner life, the life of thoughts, emotions, and physical stimuli. But we require feedback to know fully who we are to the eyes of others. In Chapters 11 and 12, awareness of inner processes is discussed in detail, but there is another side to inner awareness—the responsibility each of us has to offer feedback for others to interpret in their search for identity. We each bear a responsibility to others to offer them the opportunity to know who they are by knowing their effect upon us. Conversely, when we receive consistent criticism or praise we must listen to what is being offered as a way of assessing how our uniqueness manifests. Wishing that others would keep quiet about our foibles, or preferring not to say anything to someone with whom we have difficulty relating, prevents the exchange of feedback which offers us what the psychologist Carl Rogers calls "a soft mirror image." The key word here is "soft." Blatant complaining or a willingness to blame others entirely for relational difficulties could be the logical extreme of a willingness to offer feedback. When negative feedback masquerades as "just offering feedback" the donor soon receives feedback about being obnoxious. To be constantly critical of others demonstrates that none of the universal principles discussed so far have been taken to heart. Fault-finding with others is fault-finding with self since we all are one; it demonstrates lack of the hope implicit in knowing that everything changes, fails to recognize the complementarity of opposition, and refuses to celebrate the variety which the principle of non-duplication describes.

Faith in the intrinsic goodness, rightness, or appropriateness of where one is and what is happening, is the hallmark of spiritual leaders. This does not mean refusing to seek justice and edification in an unjust and destructive situation, but it does mean that those conditions we perceive as negative are the unique and complementary opposites of the energies we must manifest in order to effect desired change. In the recorded life of Jesus, for instance, there are numerous events in which he is anything but accepting of conditions as they exist, and he seeks, sometimes by violent means, to change them. In the process of refuting the law-based morality and religion of the Pharisees, he resorts to very strong name calling, but each confrontation is the setting for a teaching of universal truth and each proves to be the "right" setting for drawing forth the teaching. When Jesus' friend Lazarus dies, he even thanks the Father for the death since it affords opportunity to manifest the truth that there is no absolute death in this universe, that death is a change which can be changed back into life, and that "end" is a word which describes the condition which immediately precedes "beginning."

Each of us must react to those situations we encounter in our own unique way. This is why some "could care less" about issues which we consider vital, while we find it difficult to imagine how others could be so involved in issues we consider irrelevant. Thus, the principle of non-duplication also applies to perception, and it is non-duplication in perception which raises the greatest issue confronting humanity. This one world is viewed in as many ways as there are inhabitants. When groups of people gain consensus on a world view they are able to establish everything from social clubs to nations. Political ideologies, religious sects, stances on war and peace, ways of life, even ownership of a particular make of automobile is dependent upon consensus within the spectrum of unique perceptions. How often has the same movie been received with harsh criticism as well as great praise? It is the same sequence of images and the same sound effects and dialogue for all who see it, but some come away thinking that it was a terrible movie while others cannot wait to see it again.

The Gospels of the New Testament are good examples of how differently even writers attempting an historical report see events. Each Gospel was written for a specific audience and with a particular bias. The Gospel of Matthew, written by a Jew who became a Christian, was addressed to congregations of like background. For this reason Jesus is quoted as saying, "I have not come but to the lost sheep of the house of Israel," (Matthew 15:24). His ministry as fulfillment of the prophets of Jewish scriptures is alluded to constantly. Luke's Gospel has an audience of gentile Christians as its hearers composed of Greeks who were associated with Jewish houses of worship. Luke speaks their language literally and figuratively. Because of the differences in the perception of the Gospel writers, Jesus is portrayed in quite different ways in the four gospels even though the writers are believed to share common written resources as well as oral tradition. The difference between the earliest gospel, Mark, and the latest gospel, John, is really striking. As it should be in matters of faith, these differences and contradictions leave the image of the master up to the individual believer. Authorities may be appealed to, but each of us must form a unique understanding in matters of faith.

Differences in perception are the cause of what can truly be called the *problem* of good and evil. Religious writings from the earliest times have wrestled with the issues: what is good, what is evil, from whence does each come, how can we tell one from the other? The records show that there are no definitive answers to these questions outside the realm of personal belief. Many aspects of life would be much easier if the answers could be arrived at in the laboratories of science rather than in the unique crucibles of human consciousness. Those who are willing to relinquish ultimate responsibility for their beliefs and appeal to an outside authority seem blessed in regard to this *problem*. There are a multitude of such authorities, some of whose systems are very neat, offering explanations ranging from the basic depravity of human nature to the existence of two gods, one good and one evil, or to the influence of discarnate entities holding us constantly in a condition of possession by either holy spirits or evil ones.

Once there was a poor man who lived in a tiny shack with his son. He had very few possessions except a beautiful stallion which had been the gift of a Crusader who had enjoyed the ministrations and hospitality of the old man. The man was known in his village for his unwillingness to judge any situation or person. He believed and lived Jesus' injunction that we should not judge or condemn and, thereby, we would not receive ultimate judgment or condemnation. Many tried to purchase the stallion and, after each offer had been made, the old man's neighbors would ridicule his decision not to sell the horse and improve his lot with the profits. He would receive their criticisms kindly, but he considered sale of his valuable gift a betrayal of the kindness of the giver.

One day the horse escaped from his stable and ran away. Neighbors immediately descended upon the old man's hut to tell him what a fool he had been for not selling the horse while he had it. The old man's response to each visitor was the same, "Once I had the horse as a testimony to the friendship between the crusader and me; now it is gone; as to whether that is good or bad we will just have to wait to see."

In a week the stallion returned, bringing with it a herd of mares it had attracted to itself while roaming the steppes. There were eighteen of them, strong, healthy, and worth a great deal of money. The old man's neighbors flocked to his door to congratulate him on his good fortune. They were happy for him and wanted him to know how wonderful they thought this turn of events had been. The old man told each of them, "Once I had a horse; he went away; now he has returned with many horses. Whether this is good or bad we will just have to wait to see."

The son set about immediately to break the mares for saddle so that they could be sold as riding horses. The first day, he was thrown from a particularly wild one and his leg was broken. Neighbors gathered to offer condolences to the old man and his son. They were quick to offer opinions on how terrible this turn of events would prove since the old man depended so heavily on his son for maintaining their way of life. Surely this was a bad thing that had happened. The old man said, "My son has been thrown from a horse and his leg broken; as to whether or not this is a bad thing we will just have to wait to see."

Within days the king declared his country at war. Young men from all over the kingdom were conscribed for military service. Every young man in the village was taken to fight for his country except for the one with the broken leg. The old man's neighbors came in a steady stream to say how lucky he was that his son had not been taken to fight in what looked like a war which could not be won.

The truth is that at any given moment we really do not know fully whether an event is a blessing or a curse. We see only in part. Great trust in the rightness of what seems to be wrong requires vigilant discipline and really lies at the heart of spiritual work.

> Pass not judgment and you will not be judged; do not condemn and you will not be condemned; acquit and you will be acquitted; give and gifts will be given to you. Good measure, pressed down, shaken together, and running over, will be poured into your lap; for whatever measure you deal out to others will be dealt to you in return. (Luke 6:37, 38)

Sankara, the Indian saint, attained enlightenment in the marketplace near the butcher's stall. He had meditated for years and still the state of enlightenment had not come. One day, while standing in the marketplace, he overheard a conversation between a customer and the local butcher. The customer asked if she could have the butcher's best cut of meat. "All the cuts of meat here are the best!" the butcher replied. At that moment, Sankara realized that every moment was the best that it could be or it would not be at all. He ran laughing and singing back to the ashram. When his master saw him coming he knew what had happened. Sankara's joy told the story.

Joseph, the personality in the Book of Genesis whose coat of many colors has been remembered better than the events surrounding his life, was sold into slavery to the Egyptians by his jealous brothers. Joseph attained a high office in the Egyptian government and met his brothers when a famine in their country drove them to Egypt to ask for help. The story is a fascinating one and makes good reading. It can be found in Genesis, Chapters 37–50. When, at last, the brothers knew that Joseph recognized them and they were consoling each other over their father's death, they devised a means to beg Joseph's forgiveness for what they had done to him so long ago. Joseph, recognizing that many lives had been spared at the time of the famine because of his place in the government of Egypt, responded to their plea for forgiveness with, "You meant to do me harm; but God meant to bring good out of it by preserving the lives of many people, as we see today," (Genesis 50:20). Even that which is recognized by all as harmful or negative may well be only the beginning of a process which, when completed, can be assessed as good. This is because, in Ohsawa's words, "The principle of non-duplication arises because everything keeps moving toward its opposite. . . ."

Shakespeare's comment on the subject is, "Nothing is good or bad but thinking makes it so." In Paul's letter to Titus he says, "To the pure all things are pure; but nothing is pure to the tainted minds of disbelievers, tainted alike in reason and conscience," (Titus 1 : 15). In similar words he says, "I am absolutely convinced, as a Christian, that nothing is impure in itself; only, if a man considers a particular thing impure, then to him it is impure," (Romans 14 : 14).[2] George Ohsawa says of good and evil, "On earth we call 'good' what we like, and 'evil' what we do not like—what we conceive to be helpful to man and what we consider to be harmful. What is good for one man, however, may be harmful for another. Virtues, under certain circumstances, may appear as vices—as when thrift becomes stinginess, courage rashness, patience lethargy."[3]

In a commentary on good and evil which encompasses several of the principles being considered here, Ohsawa says, "According to the Unique Principle, neither good nor evil exist; only yin and yang, antagonistic and complementary. All that is antagonistic is complementary and indispensable, each to the other . . . in this world of relativity, everything changes, turning into opposite extremes. One may then say that that which is eternal, absolute and infinite is the only *good* and that which is not absolute, infinite, or eternal is the only *evil*."[4] The third Chinese Patriarch of Zen, called Sosan in Japan, said, "The Great Way is not difficult for those who have no preferences. Make the smallest distinction, however, and heaven and earth are set infinitely apart. If you wish to see the truth then hold no opinions for or against anything. . . . Indeed, it is in our choosing to accept or reject that we do not see the true nature of things."

In a world which might be stopped and examined, we would be able to isolate the good and the evil according to our own value system. A static world does not exist, however, and in the flow of events, in accordance with the law of change, what was evil becomes good, what was good becomes a bane to our existence. Art Buchwald captures this flow with hilarious precision in a description of a conversation with his son following a trip to the movies where they saw *The Battle of The Coral Sea*. After leaving the theater, they discussed the film at a sidewalk cafe:

> At the table he said to me: "The Japanese were very bad people to do those things to the Americans, weren't they?"
> "Yes," I said, "but they're not bad people now."
> "Why?" he wanted to know.
> "Because they don't do things like that any more."
> He thought about this a minute and then said: "Why did they do all those bad things then?"
> "Probably they didn't know they were doing bad things. They probably thought they were doing good things."
> "Why didn't someone tell them?" he wanted to know.
> "We tried," I said, "but they wouldn't listen."
> "Remember that war picture we saw some weeks ago? The one about the Germans and how they beat the poor people and the children in the prison camp?"
> "Yes," I said.
> "The Germans are bad people, aren't they?"
> "No," I said. "They *were* bad people, but now they're good people."
> "Are they different people?" he wanted to know.
> "No, they're the same people. At least many are the same people. You see, once you fight a war you can't stay mad at the people after the war is over. You have to forget what the bad people did during the war, because if you don't there could be another war."
> "But in the movies they're still bad people," he said.
> "Yes, that's to remind us that they were bad people, but we're supposed to forget it."
> He looked at me blankly.
> "Did you kill any Russians during the war?" he wanted to know a few minutes later.
> "No. Because during the war they were good people and

they fought the Germans just like the British and Americans did."

"But if they were good people during the war and killed the bad people, why are they bad people now?"

"They're not bad now. Most of the Russians are good people. But we don't agree with what their leaders say and want to do. And they don't agree with us. That's why we're having trouble in Germany."

"With the bad Germans?"

"No, with the good Germans. The bad Germans want to kick the good Germans out of Berlin."

"Then there are still bad Germans?"

"Yes, but there are also good Germans. You see, after the war the country was divided and the Russians occupied half of it and we occupied the other half."

"Why didn't the Russians kill the bad Germans, if they were bad?"

"Well, the Russians don't think their Germans are bad. They think their Germans are good. They think our Germans are bad. We think their Germans, at least their German leaders, are bad, and our Germans are good. You understand?"

He said, "No."

"Well, it doesn't make any difference if you understand it or not," I said angrily, "Everyone else does. I never saw a kid who asked so many silly questions."[5]

Serious work has been done by immunerable theologians and scholars on the problem of good and evil. Highly complex systems of thought, bringing into play the full range of cognitive faculties, have been devised to resolve the questions posed by the existence of the negative in a creation differentiating from one infinity, an infinity held to be all good—all God. However, there is no simpler statement of the truth which resolves this issue than that in The Book of Lamentations:

> Who has commanded and it came to pass, unless the Lord has ordained it? Is it not from the mouth of the Most High that good and evil come? (Lamentations 3:37, 38)

It would be unfair to such an important subject to leave the reader with a few anecdotes and a Bible quote as the total discussion. The way evil sneaks into the best of situations was recognized by the writer of the Garden of Eden myth, and the serpent, that slithering creature, was chosen to personalize it. In eating from the tree (there's no mention of apples) Adam and Eve lost their consciousness of the undifferentiated One and began to make distinctions. They attained awareness of "this and that," the knowledge of good and evil. Had Sosan been around, he could have told them why they recognized their differences, their nakedness. They had exercised their privilege as creatures created in the image of the creator. They had created, too. They had chosen to do something which their creator had asked them not to do, and had begun creating their own reality; it was painful.

The third chapter of Genesis contains this story, written 2,900 years ago and filled with truths which still resonate today. Some take the story literally while others understand it as the work of a master storyteller demonstrating universal truths not to be taken as historical and scientific fact. Whatever the interpretation, the universal truths are there and each of us is East of Eden, caught up in discriminating between this and that, judging, condemning, and attempting to get back to that state where we could walk with God "in the cool of the evening" (Genesis 3:8) without the nagging knowledge of good and evil. It is the purpose of the macrobiotic way of life to enable that return by curing the arrogance which sees only separateness and facilitating the ascending spiral of creation back to the undifferentiated One. That is the macrobiotic way of saying that, through appropriate diet, attention to spiritual development, and a natural lifestyle, we are enabled to realize our place in the Kingdom of Heaven.

The Eden incident is known, theologically, as "the Fall." It is considered to be the moment when humankind fell from grace, willingly separated ourselves from God, and stood in need of redemption. This traditional interpretation of the beginning of good and evil has stood for two millennia in Christian circles where theologians and believers posit Jesus as the "second Adam" who redeems us from this separation from God, undoing what was done by the first Adam. Matthew Fox, in his interpretation, echoes the growing understanding that the Eden scene is not the occasion of original sin but original blessing and has so titled his book, *Original Blessing*. It is this very ability to choose between good and evil which makes us human, allows for creative possibilities, and generates both the agony and the ecstasy which gives a vivifying dynamic to human life. Rather than seeing humanity as sinful, a creation-centered theology sees us as divine but capable of demonic and sinful choices. In the fall/redemption theology, emphasis is on Jesus as the Son of God while, in Fox's view, he is also prophet, artist, and parable-teller who calls others to their divinity. He is the quintessential celebrant of life who calls us to follow him in celebration made possible by radical trust in the infinite goodness of the Father within. The first chapter of the Bible, the story of creation, ends with the words, "And God saw everything that he had made and it was very Good," (Genesis 1:31). These are very ancient words, driven deep in the understanding of the culture out of which they were penned three millennia ago. We still have not taken them to heart. We question their veracity by making judgments and distinctions, and we have trouble letting go and falling into total trust.

One day a jogger fell into a ravine. He managed to grab a tree on the way down to certain death. The bottom lay a hundred feet below him. He began to scream, "Is there anybody up there?" Perhaps a passerby would hear him and summon help. "Is there anybody up there?" he screamed over and over again. Just when his strength was failing, a loud and resonant voice filled the ravine. It seemed to emanate from the rocks themselves, and it said, "You are not alone! I am with you. You will be delivered safely to the bottom. Let go of the branch and you will float down to safety borne on the wings of my love." The jogger thought a minute then screamed, "Is there anybody *else* up there?"

Dr. H. Emilie Cady, in her book, *Lessons in Truth,* says, "The very circumstances in your life that seem heartbreaking evils will turn to joy before your very eyes if you will steadfastly refuse to see anything but God in them"[6] The work to which each of us is called is to take responsibility for creating the physical, mental, and spiritual condition which enables us to have eyes to see and ears to hear this truth.

The history of consideration of the problem posed by good and evil is covered in detail in the book, *Evil and The God of Love,* by John Hick. He traces the history of theological discussion in Christian circles in a manner which makes his book a valuable reference for any reader wishing more serious study than can be offered in these pages.

An area of special interest in the context of both macrobiotics and the Christian faith which demonstrates forcefully the principle of non-duplication is that of healing and disease. The occurrence of what is recognized clinically as the same disease shows tremendous variation from person to person. It becomes obvious when dealing with numbers of patients why healing is truly described as an art rather than a science. Each illness is peculiar to the sufferer. When a person describes an illness as, "My arthritis," or "My heart trouble," they have identified both a part of the problem and a key to its solution. Our unique states of imbalance manifest in unique ways. Each requires unique treatment designed to meet each personal need. When disease becomes an important part of a person's identity, as so often happens with degenerative diseases, the onset of which takes many years, a cure cannot be effected without a change in identity. It is frightening to many to contemplate an identity change and, therefore, long-term diseases may be exceedingly stubborn. The real concern, then, is with the person rather than with the broad category of the particular disease. The principle of non-duplication should serve as a constant reminder to set categories aside and deal with each unique particularity. This approach avoids the dehumanizing effect of relegating real people to arbitrary categories and recognizes the validity of each person's needs. This attitude is an intrinsic part of both macrobiotic and Christian approaches to healing. As with all events in our lives, disease arises as part of our learning and growth. It is an offering from which we are to benefit. George Ohsawa states:

> If any illness is sent to us, it is meant as a warning, an alarm signal. Illness is not sent to us as a punishment, but as a final offering of saving grace. We have only to pay heed to our bodies to know what we must do.[7]

Seeing disease as good may seem heresy to those whose lack of trust in the basic goodness of creation causes perceptions of negativity. It is not unusual to find patients today who believe that their disease is a punishment. They still have not learned the lesson understood by early second century Christians whose Church produced the Gospel of John. These early believers report Jesus' response to the question of punishment in this way:

> As he went on his way Jesus saw a man blind from his birth. His disciples put the question, "Rabbi, who sinned, this man or his parents? Why was he born blind?" "It is not that this man or his parents sinned," Jesus answered; "He was born blind that God's power might be displayed in curing him." (John 9: 1–3)

Disease comes as an opportunity rather than a curse, a warning rather than a punishment, a call to wholeness rather than a death sentence.

Personal responsiblity in creating the conditions which allow healing to take place is also a common theme in macrobiotics and Christianity. Michio Kushi states:

> When we are in misery, it is caused by our wrong judgment, which may come from a way of life out of harmony with the

> environment. Sickness, accident, miseries and any other difficulties can be turned to health, well-being and happiness through only a change of our own thought and conduct. No one else can change them on our behalf—we must initiate change ourselves. We may receive advice, suggestions and guidance, but it is we who should act as the masters of our own destiny.[8]

This is reminiscent of Paul's advice to "work out our own salvation," and Jesus' admonition to "take up your cross and follow me." The Rev. Dr. John Ruef paraphrases this quote from Jesus as, "Take on your you-ness."[9]

Just as the manifestation of a disease is unique to us, so only by our unique response to it can healing be effected. In Christian terms, that unique response is our own response of faith—faith in the healing method, faith in the basic goodness of the disease event, faith in wholeness as the ultimate state of creation, faith in the irresistible grace of God to whom all things are possible. Jesus lays this responsibility upon those he heals when time after time healing events are followed with the words, "Your faith has cured you," or "Your faith has made you whole." Often these words are followed by, "Go, sin no more." Sin is understood here in its true sense of simply missing the mark, not being in harmony with the order of the universe, a sense of separation or arrogance.[10] Jesus recognized personal responsibility both for the healing at the moment and the way of life to be followed in the future to prevent future disease.

The macrobiotic way is the way of the whole of life; it is the large view of the universe and our place in it. It is a wholistic approach. Parts of the disease process may be analyzed and assessed for their contributory nature, but only as those parts make up the whole can any disease or imbalance be treated. The whole is greater than the sum of the parts. These days holistic health centers, holistic therapies and therapists seem to be nothing new. New age publications and even more traditional journals stress the importance of considering the whole life in treating physical and emotional difficulties. This growing recognition of the truth of an orderly universe of mutually interdependent parts is not a recent discovery but, rather, a recent recovery of the ancient understanding that the universe is one.

It should come as no surprise that one of the greatest healers who ever lived, Jesus of Nazareth, practiced a wholistic approach. Thanks to our Western Germanic linguistic roots we can trace the words "whole," "heal," "health," and "holy" back to the same word. The wholistic approach is truly the holy one. Jesus did not attempt to explain disease, but his attitude toward it shows a marked difference from that of the Old Testament in which disease is seen as punishment and looked upon with contempt. His ministry is closely bound up with the sick and feeble of body and soul. The pages of the Gospels are filled with stories of healings, as his reputation, and people's faith in the possibility of wholeness, grew. Since he viewed the individual as an essential unity of body and mind, he invariably paid close attention to the mind and spirit of the sufferer. This attitude stands in stark opposition to the Greek view that the body was the prison house of the soul.[11] In the several detailed accounts of interviews with sufferers, Jesus is portrayed as attempting to uncover evidence that disease is an aspect of a deficient relationship between the sufferer and total environment. His encounter with the Samaritan woman at the well in John 4, becomes a powerful therapeutic analysis revealing chaos and conflict in her personal life.

In his teaching, Jesus' attitude toward the importance of deep workings of the inner mind is revealed. His ministry was as much to the mind as the body. The Sermon on the Mount, in Matthew 5, deals with emotional conflict, fear, resentment, anxiety, and hatred, all of which are stress factors with the power to produce a radical imbalance capable of promoting organic damage. The fact that we can blush in embarrassment should be all we need to know regarding the effect of emotional values on the physiology of the body. When a far more serious trauma than simple embarrassment is exprerienced the effects can be devastating. Lawrence LeShan's work in developing a profile for the cancer-prone personality shows that loss of a crucial relationship, inability to express hostility, and tension over the death of a parent are three among several stress factors found in cancer patients. In one study, LeShan found that 72 percent of the cancer patients interviewed had experienced the loss of a crucial relationship.[12] This statistic sheds an interesting light on Jesus' constant concern with love of neighbor, willingness to share, freedom from judging, and lack of possessiveness as they relate to wholeness. The roots of psychogenic disease lie very deep in the human personality; so do the roots of faith, hope, and love.

Each sufferer was treated in a unique way by Jesus, sometimes with a word, a touch, through the faith of others, by making a compress out of mud with spittle,[13] or even with a "loud cry" as in the raising of Lazarus. This tells us that Jesus had assessed the person's condition correctly and was aware of the factors which had contributed to its incidence. He had performed a "consultation" and had used his powers of diagnosis. No two diseases were seen to be alike. Each person was healed in his own way by his own faith and will to live.

Michio Kushi cites five factors which may be indicators of terminality in a diseased person: arrogance, inaccuracy in life style, no will to live, no family support, loss of natural healing ability due to radical medical procedures. Three of these factors are psychological/emotional with aspects of "inaccuracy in life style" falling into this category. The American Cancer Society claims that 90 percent of all cancers are caused by environmental factors. Surely the inner environment of mind and spirit must be included along with the air we breathe and the food we eat.

George Ohsawa defines health as freedom from fatigue, good appetite, sound sleep, good memory, good humor, and precision in thought and action.[14] Three are physical; three are psychological. Together they describe a person with dynamism, joy, intelligence, clear conscience, and sound judgment. The world is in desperate need of those who bear the wisdom to create such conditions in themselves. The macrobiotic way of life, in its concern for the whole person, offers the possibility of attaining this wisdom. Dietary guidelines, emphasis on physical exercise, and encouragement of a gratitude-filled, active life of faith forms the basis of the macrobiotic understanding of the needs of a whole human being, and produces wisdom intrinsic in human nature which need only be uncovered and reclaimed.

Late in the Old Testament period and during the intertestamental times, wisdom was recognized as emanating from the creator as a first act of creation. It was personalized, interestingly enough and thanks to the Greeks, in the feminine gender, and, in what is known as wisdom literature, elevated to a status virtually equal with God. The playful delight which wisdom manifests in the following quote from Proverbs 8, has the ring of macrobiotic literature and is included here as a strikingly poetic description of the wisdom we seek.

> Hear how Wisdom lifts her voice and Understanding cries out . . . The Lord created me in the beginning of his works, before all else that he made long ago. Alone, I was fashioned in times long past, at the beginning, long before earth itself. When there was yet no ocean I was born, no springs brimming with water. Before mountains were settled in their place, long before the hills I was born, when as yet he had made neither land nor lake nor the first clod of earth. When he set the heavens in their place I was there, when he girdled the ocean with the horizon, when he fixed the canopy of clouds overhead and set the springs of ocean firm in their place, when he prescribed its limits for the sea and knit together earth's foundations. I was at his side each day, his darling and delight, playing in his presence continually, playing on earth when he had finished it, while my delight was in mankind.
>
> Now my sons, listen to me, listen to instruction and grow wise, do not reject it. Happy is the one who keeps to my ways, happy the one who listens to me, watching daily at my threshold with his eyes on the doorway; for he who finds me finds life and wins favor with the Lord, while he who finds

me not hurts himself, and all who hate me are in love with death. (Proverbs 8 : 1, 22–36)

From the Didache echoes:

There are two ways: the way of life and the way of death.

---

[1] *Macromuse*, issue number 15, quotation from *Book of Judo*, by George Ohsawa, Chapter 9.
[2] This quote refers specifically to food which had been offered to idols.
[3] Ohsawa, *You are All Sanpaku*, p. 87.
[4] Ohsawa, *The Book of Judgment*, pp. 103–104.
[5] Buchwald, *Down The Seine and Up The Potomac*, pp. 26, 27.
[6] Cady, *Lessons in Truth*, p. 15.
[7] Ohsawa, *You are All Sampaku*, p. 77.
[8] Kushi, *The Book of Macrobiotics*, p. 96.
[9] Ruef, *Understanding The Gospels*, p. 61.
[10] The Biblical use of the word "sin" in both Hebrew and Greek means "to miss." There is no implication of guilt-ridden breast-beating.
[11] Descartes, in a much later period, likewise divided the person into physical, *substantia extensa*, and the mental, *substantia cogitans*, categories. Descartes believed the latter to be the proper domain of the Church.
[12] LeShan, *You Can Fight For Your Life*, p. 26.
[13] Spittle was understood, in Jesus time, to contain the vital energies of the person. As the sign of the cross replaced that of the fish in the early Church and people "crossed themselves," that act is reported to have been done on the forehead with the thumb moistened with spit.
[14] Ohsawa, *You are All Sampaku*, pp. 62–64.

Chapter 5

What has a Front has a Back, The Bigger the Front the Bigger the Back

"Blessed are the poor in spirit, for theirs is the Kingdom of Heaven." (Matthew 5:3)

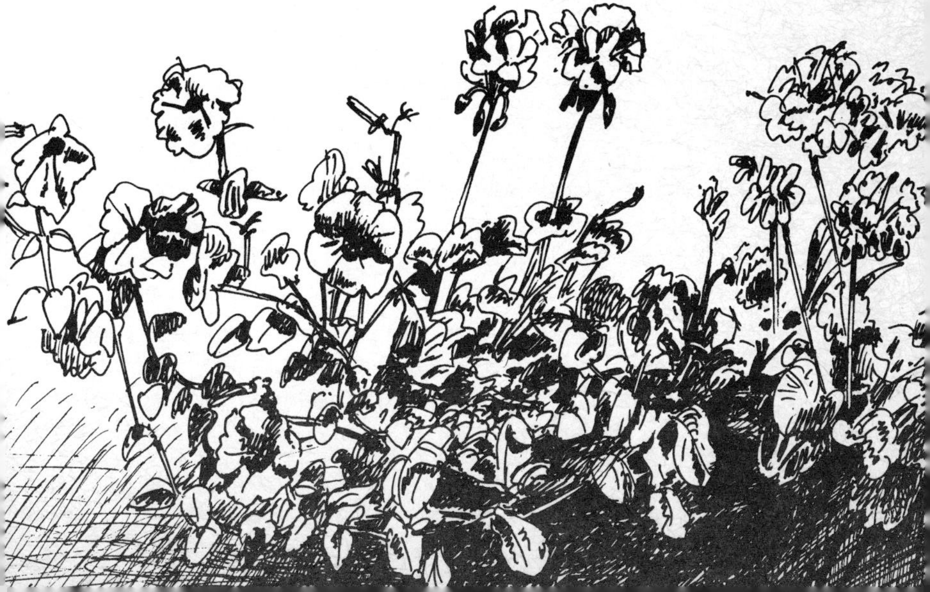

THE TWO PRINCIPLES DESCRIBING THE UNIVERSAL OCCURRENCE of fronts and backs and their proportional relationship will be considered together in this chapter. These principles are, so to speak, both sides of the "both sides" issue. They mark a distinct change in the tone of the list of principles and sound almost too simple to be included in a list of universals. Everyone knows that every front has a back or it couldn't be a front. What, then, do these principles mean, and how do they apply in daily life? Why are they important enough to be included in a list of only seven universals?

The Seven Principles of The Infinite Universe describe an ever-changing unity, no two parts of which are identical and all opposing parts being complementary. Each part of this unity manifests with a front and back of matching proportions, and everything with a beginning has an end. These things with matching fronts and backs are described by the first four principles as unique, constantly changing constellations of creative energy which express One, infinite source and, when confronted by antagonistic opposition, that opposition is seen to be an integral part of the identity of both opposites.

Since these princples are universals, they are universally manifesting and it is impossible to isolate operation of one of the principles without considering the other principles which are also at work. Fronts and backs are differentiations of one infinity, changing even as they are examined. They are opposing, therefore non-identical, sides of the manifestation they comprise, and eventually they will cease to be, since they had a beginning. The principles under discussion are a further description of principle three—all anatgonisms are complementary. In these principles we see that all antagonisms are also necessary, that everything comes in two's with a front and a back, a proponent and an opponent, a high and a low, a night and a day, matter and anti-matter. If there is a Winter, there will be a Summer, if a mountain, then a valley. In short, as soon as anything manifests this side of the Undifferentiated One, its opposite also manifests, or there could be no manifestation at all.

In applying these principles to proponents and opponents of an issue a number of interesting observations arise. First, it becomes obvious that the fronts and backs principles apply to more than just quantitative factors but also include qualities, such as political power. One proponent with political power may successfully oppose the desires of many opponents without power. Intensity of feeling can also be a compensating quality since a few highly motivated people can work their wills over the many who are only half-heartedly in opposition.

Secondly, each proponent and opponent also has a front and a back. Just as each issue is given its identity by those who compose its front and back, its pro's and con's, so each proponent is a potential opponent of equivalent intensity. Great saints are aware of their potential to become great sinners, the *nouveau riche* is in danger of sudden poverty, today's superstar can be tomorrow's has-been. The other side of the previous three comparisons is that great sinners have the potential to become great saints, the poor to become rich, and the unknown to be catapulted into great publicity.

Thirdly, since fronts and backs compose the whole, both hope and the danger of unfulfilled expectations exist in every situation. The torrid romance can grow very cold, the unrewarding relationship become fulfilling, the threat of immanent divorce become the key to the kind of open communication which keeps a marriage vital.

Principle two, everything changes, works with the principles of fronts and backs as the cause of both the hope and the anguish. Things are changing into their opposites. When "this, too" passes, it passes into its opposite. This fact is the origin of the expression, "shirtsleeves to shirtsleeves in three generations" as a poor family becomes wealthy and the wealth is squandered and lost by subsequent generations. At the 1983 North American Macrobiotic Congress, Lima Ohsawa made an impassioned plea for marital fidelity and reconciliation based on the interaction of principles two, five and six and the hope for the future which that interaction implies.

Since the universal principles describe all that is, they are operating all the time. Knowledge of them can be deepened and internalized by looking to them to describe any situation or personal condition. This practice will soon make the principles come alive with meaning reflecting the subtle shadings of their interaction. They are, truly, "the law of the Lord" in that they describe the workings of creation. By following their simple logic, the order of the universe can be applied for health and happiness. This and seemingly more extravagant claims have been made by George Ohsawa, and those claims are true. Just how true they are cannot be appreciated until we become like the person who is blessed because "his delight is in the law of the Lord, and in his law doth he meditate day and night," (Psalm 1:2). Practice seeing the back which is the other side of the front of any situation for a few days and deeper understanding will come very quickly.

The two principles which are the subject of this chapter must have been considered of tremendous importance by George Ohsawa. They comprise two sevenths of his list of universal laws, and first exist in the form we find them in an early work, *The Book of Judo* published in 1952. Other principles were changed, verbally, before attaining final form as we have them and being listed as an annex to the "Constitution of the Eternal World Peace" published in 1966. Fortunately, they are among the easiest to see and to understand although all of the principles are natural and, therefore, none should be difficult. If there is difficulty in understanding the principles, it is the difficulty which attends the understanding of all universal truth: making the transition from head to heart. That is why so many saints and mystics refer to their spiritual discipline or sadhana as "the work." The work which attends any way of life is to *do it*. Our work is to experience, consciously, "the laws of God" in operation, to wake up, to be aware.

As practice, let us look at the front and the back of a biblical character whose two sides are exceedingly obvious—Saul of Tarsus, persecutor of the early church, who became its first and greatest theologian. Paul was trained by Gamaliel, the man who advised his fellow Jewish rulers not to deal harshly with the followers of Jesus because if what the early church was doing was not "of God" then it would pass away, and if "of God" anyone opposing it would be "at war with God," (Acts 5:39). He was a wise man and, perhaps, the seed of his deep faith in the justice of God without the necessity of human intervention was planted in his young student only to blossom on the road to Damascus. It was at Paul's feet that those who killed the first Christian martyr, St. Stephen, laid their coats. Paul was rigid, a Pharisee for whom life was to be lived according to every detail of the law. The Pharisees were the group who constantly confronted Jesus with questions about why he and his disciples did not observe one regulation or another. These laws were akin to canon law in the church, intramural issues of interpretation of universal truths many times removed from the beauty and the simplicity of Jesus' summary of the law: love of God and love of neighbor as self. In retribution for the blasphemous claim that Jesus was the Messiah, Paul, then known as Saul, sought the imprisonment and extermination of all Christians.

Paul came by his zeal and rigidity naturally. We know that he was raised in Tarsus of Cilicia, a Greek-speaking city. He was the son of Jewish parents who had made their home in that alien land. There were Jewish communities in all of the important cities of the Roman empire. Their residents either had been carried off as slaves or were drawn by opporunities for trade. Worship was essentially home-based, with regular gatherings at synagogues for prayer and study of The Law and The Prophets. This worship took place in cities festooned with statues and symbols of other religions. One had to cling tenaciously to one's own faith not to be swayed by so many other possibilities for religious expression. Saul was of a small minority group in a pagan city.

His secondary education (as we would call it) took place in Jerusalem at Gamaliel's academy, completion of which made him one of the best educated men of his time and marked him out as a young man with a future. Looking back on those days he writes,

"I was forging ahead in Judaism, beyond many of my own age among my people—I was so full of zeal for the traditions of my fathers," (Galatians 1:14). Those traditions were threatened by the followers of Jesus, and Paul's zeal was given life by what he saw as antagonistic to his religion.

The story of Paul's one hundred eighty degree turn of consciousness, when he turned back to front, is recounted in the following words:

> Meanwhile Saul was still breathing murderous threats against the disciples of the Lord. He went to the High Priest and applied for letters to the synagogues at Damascus authorizing him to arrest anyone he found, men or women, who followed the new way, and bring them to Jerusalem. While he was still on the road and nearing Damascus, suddenly a light flashed from the sky all around him. He fell to the ground and heard a voice saying, "Saul, Saul, why do you persecute me?" "Tell me, Lord," he said, "who are you?" "I am Jesus, whom you are persecuting." (Acts 9: 1–5)

Paul was left blinded by the event, proceeded to Damascus, and there was healed of his blindness by a disciple named Ananias after three days of fasting. He was baptized and from that day on became a devoted Christian, producing what is the earliest writing in the New Testament, and the theology which became the foundation for all later Christian understanding. His writing is difficult, and he has been much maligned, especially when taken out of cultural context. Some of his teaching is based upon the erroneous notion of Jesus' immediate return, in the flesh, during the lifetimes of some of his contemporaries. When Paul's teaching on marriage only as a last resort (1 Corinthians 7:9), for instance, is read with this in mind it makes such a statement understandable. Why plan to get married if the end of the age may be here at any second?

Paul's front of intense zeal and fanatical devotion to the traditions of his fathers was matched by a back of equal proportions, one of immovable conviction of the truth of Jesus' messiahship and of the "unsearchable riches" (Ephesians 3:8) which that conviction conveys—the very "way" originally he sought to eradicate! In Paul's experiences we encounter the true meaning of conversion: "turning," or "returning." It is the familiar word, "conversion," which describes so well the turning from front to back, that flip-flop of consciousness which is so sudden as to seem surprisingly unnatural, even supernatural. The word for "conversion" in both Hebrew and Greek carries the above meaning and occurs frequently in the Old Testament. As a noun, it occurs only once in the New Testament, in Acts 15:3, in the reference to the "conversion of the Gentiles." The Children of Israel are admonished: "Return to me, apostate children, says the Lord, for I am patient with you . . ." (Jeremiah 3:14), and they implore, "O Lord, turn us back to thyself and we will come back," in Lamentations 5:21. The theology of the latter quote recognizes the unity of creation, the truth that when creation acts, it acts because the creator is acting through it. Conversion is not only a turning toward the creator, but can be a turning away as well: "Then why are this people so wayward, incurable in their waywardness? Why have they clung to their treachery and refused to *return* to their obedience?" (Jeremiah 8:5), and "As soon as Gideon died, the people of Israel *turned again* and played the harlot after the Baals, and made Baal-berith their God," Judges 8:33). In the New testament, this turning away appears as well: "But now that you do acknowledge God—or rather, now that he has acknowledged you—how can you turn back to the mean and beggarly spirits of the elements?" (Galatians 4:9). The most characteristic use of conversion is as a turning toward God, whether or not there had ever been a conscious turning away. The people of the towans of Lydda and Sharon, at seeing Aeneas cured, "turned to the Lord" (Acts 9:35b). Sometimes the nature of the turning is described as in Acts 26:18—from darkness to light, or 1 Thessalonians 1:9—from idols to God, or Acts 14:15—from vain things to a living God. Paul even describes what is effected by the turning as "the veil is removed," (2 Corinthians 3: 16) which would certainly result in someone having "seen the light." This leads Paul, in a subsequent verse to say, "And because for us there is no veil over the face, we all reflect as in a mirror the splendor of the Lord; thus we are transfigured into his likeness, from splendor to splendor; such is the influence of the Lord who is spirit," (2 Corinthians 3: 18). In macrobiotic rhetoric, this certainly is a description of the result of ascending the spiral of creation. To turn one's consciousness from front to back or from back to front, to experience "conversion," is at the heart of the Church's earliest recorded injunctions. "Repent, and believe the Gospel," (Mark 1: 15) is a call to turn from the way of death, to recognize that the front of resistance contains its complementary, opposite back of equivalent proportion through conversion to the way of life.

One of the least likely New Testament candidates for vacillation is that rocky personality, Peter. His name was Simon, but Jesus called him Peter as a nickname best translated into English as "Rocky." Jesus even says, "Upon this rock will I build my Church," (Matthew 16: 18). Peter was among the first disciples called to follow Jesus, and was one of the three closest associates whose name, along with James and John, appears in connection with the major events of Jesus' life. He was of the inner circle and is identified as the one who confessed to Jesus that he believed him to be the anointed One, or Messiah. Paul refers to Peter as Cephus, or "head" of the early Christian community. This man was obviously devoted to his master, having left all he owned to follow him, and had witnessed events which should leave anyone convinced of the authenticity of Jesus' unity with the Father. Yet, when Jesus says that he must suffer and be killed Peter actually laid hold of him, taking him by the arm, and rebuked him. When Jesus asked Peter, James, and John to be with him during his trying moments in the Garden of Gethsemane, Peter and the others fell asleep while their master is described as literally sweating blood (Luke 22: 44). Matthew even adds that Jesus had to wake them up three times, asking them each time if they could not even stay awake with him for this ordeal. Finally, Peter denies knowing Jesus, as was predicted by the master, in a scene in a courtyard outside the place where Jesus was on trial the night before he was killed. Yet, Peter was one of the first at the tomb on the day of the resurrection and one of the first to believe in the reality of that event. He may well set the record for front to back flip-flops among the New Testament characters. It was not until the day of Pentecost, some fifty days after the resurrection, that the stability of Peter's faith was assured and his predicted rock-like leadership established in the biblical record.

Although Peter's vacillation may seem like the least likely to have occurred, our understanding that every front has a back of like proportion would predict such a possibility. The back side of faith is doubt. Indeed, there cannot be one without the other. Faith is a universal in world religions and so there are stories of faith and doubt in the literature of them all. Faith in the Buddha's enlightenment is often described as being accompanied by a "ball of doubt.' The law of change advises us that everything is changing into its opposite, including faith into doubt and doubt into faith. The issue for the believer is how to keep one's consciousness fixed upon faith rather than becoming fixated upon growing doubt when it arises. The greatest New Testament example of doubt followed by faith is found in Thomas the doubter, whose name is still associated with his former state rather than the latter. His doubt in Jesus' resurrection was so great that he required a physical examination of the master's wounds before he would believe. This story, reported only by John in Chapter 20, verse 27, may not be historic fact since the other writers do not include it, but it does represent the truth of the front and back of doubt and faith. Its inclusion is a striking embellishment of the human traits exhibited by those first and closest followers of Jesus at a time when they were obviously confused and frightened by the events of the few days past.

Saints have reported periods of their lives when only the "ball of doubt" seemed to manifest. These times have been called "dry periods" when the water of the Spirit seemed not to flow. Yet, these times passed, as any student of the seven universal principles and/or reader of the Bible knows they must. The attitude which makes these times tolerable for the believer must be one of clinging to whatever faith may be there, even if it is only the size of a mustard seed, until it follows the inexorable law of change and grows into something more substantial. This may have to be accomplished by an act of will rather than as the natural flowering of the well-watered seed. Such an act can prevent what both the Old and New Testament call "double-mindedness," that wavering condition between faith and doubt which prevents the object of prayer from manifesting. The Epistle of James recommends that the believer "ask in faith, without a doubt in his mind; for the doubter is like the heaving sea ruffled by the wind. A man of that kind must not expect the Lord to give him anything; he is double-minded, and never can keep a steady course," (James 1:7, 8). This approach does not disallow the existence of doubt, but only that the doubt not be vivified by being given conscious credence. It means keeping the eye single (Matthew 6:22) and not serving two masters (Matthew 6:24). It means having "faith and no doubts," a state in which mountains can be moved; and whatever is prayed for will be received, (Matthew 21:21, 22). It is not faith which needs assistance but the lack of it, so that the existence of doubt will be driven from awareness. After Jesus heals the boy made speechless and driven to grand mal seizures by spirit possession, he tells the boy's father, "Everything is possible to one who has faith." "I believe," cries the father, "help my unbelief," (Mark 9:23, 24). We do not need help with faith; faith creates its own reinforcement; it is doubt that we need help overcoming.

Faith, whether defined in traditional biblical terms or as George Ohsawa does, (as understanding the unique principle, the divine economy), requires some change of outer behavior as well as inner attitude to be genuine. When the front disappears and the back manifests there is a change in consciousness which results in a change in life style. Sometimes it is the change in behavior which signals that the inner change has occurred. A realization that one is not as judgmental as in the past means that the truth of the unity of creation is beginning to dawn. There has been a change in attitude, a heightened realization of the unity which, in fact, we share as creatures of one creative power. The Epistle of James states, ". . . by my deeds I will prove to you my faith," and "faith divorced from deeds is barren," (James 2: 19, 21). The following statement on faith and works, in this letter to early believers, is a fine statement to all of us who profess to follow a way of life and yet forget the life-giving actions which are required for authenticity: "My brothers, what use is it for a man to say that he has faith when he does nothing to show it? Can faith save him? Suppose a brother or a sister is in rags with not enough food for the day, and one of you says, 'Good luck to you, keep yourselves warm and have plenty to eat,' but does nothing to supply their bodily needs, what is the good of that? So with faith; if it does not lead to action, it is in itself a lifeless thing." (James 2: 14–17). It is not what we say we believe that describes our faith but how we live our lives.

People of true power are those whose inner convictions, their faith and understanding, is translated directly into action which mirrors those convictions. The saints canonized by the church are such people. Had they been presented with the list of the seven principles, their response might well have been, "Of course!" Rather than what James calls "barren," their faith resulted in the birth of countless good works and inspirations which still move the faithful. Saint. Francis of Assisi was such a person; he is so loved and admired that other religions claim him as one of theirs because he manifested the universal spirit of truth in his simplicity and devotion, in his joy and celebration, in his extreme pain and mortification. He lived both sides of the human condition and celebrated them with equal intensity. His interest in all of creation reflected an interest in the creator. He referred to everything, from the sun to the cauterizing iron about to be placed on his eyes, as "brother." He called the moon and the birds who became silent at his bidding his "sisters." Francis lived the belief that this universe is a differentiation of one infinity in whose life we participate:

> What gave him his extraordinary personal power was this: that from the Pope to the beggar, from the sultan of Syria in his pavilion to the ragged robbers crawling out of the woods, there was never a man who looked into those brown burning eyes without being certain that Francis Bernardone was really interested in *him*; in his own inner individual life from the cradle to the grave; that he himself was being valued and taken seriously, and not merely added to the spoils of some social policy or the names in some clerical document."[1]

Francis was simply living out the injunction of the Master whom Francis believed to be the incarnation of the One: "Inasmuch as you have done it to one of the least of these my brethren you have done it unto me," (Matthew 25:40). For him, the creator was what one modern writer has called "our touchable Lord."

When given an opportunity to run its course behavior which tends toward disintegration—destructive, non-edifying, self-sabotaging behavior—can die of its own accord. It can spin itself out and result in the realization that the other side of that behavior is all that is left to us—the integrative, constructive, self-affirming action. An old and wise member of my family has suggested an admittedly simplistic solution to the drug problem. His suggestion is that the government construct an enormous compound where anyone convicted of drug-related offenses would be placed and given a steady diet of whatever drugs they prefer until they become so sick of it all that they drop the attachment and reenter society. This same approach is advocated by the Indian spiritual leader Rajneesh, whose application of it to misdirected sensuality and egoism has resulted in worldwide bad press and misunderstanding. Many group activities sponsored by his followers encourage wallowing in sensuality and egoism, awaiting the day when it will drop of its own accord rather than be repressed only to resurface and have to be dealt with all over again. Backs and fronts must be present together. The question is how to short-circuit attachment to and identification with the dark side so that the light may shine through us.

Whether or not attachment to the one side dies, so that faith in the power of the positive manifests in a change of life, depends upon a host of factors. The most important is how much one's personal identity depends upon that particular facet of life. If identity is virtually totally dependent upon a certain thing, regardless of how irrelevant and inconsequential that thing may seem to a disinterested observer, that person may, and in some cases actually elects to, die rather than change it. Such cases are seen regularly by macrobiotic counselors regarding attachment to certain dietary patterns which have been instrumental in the onset of disease. Many people in the chronological prime of life actually would rather die than change their diet. A man in my home town always drove a Cadillac. He was not a man of means, but insisted on that particular make of automobile. As the years went by and his cars disintegrated he purchased vehicles succeedingly more used until, for the same price, he could have had a far newer and more attractive Chevrolet, but he drove his junker Cadillac until one finally outlived him.

The following is one of the most famous New Testament stories which contains not only a demonstration of the front and back principles but an example of how change of attitude, change of behavior, and the redirecting of consciousness leads to the way of life rather than the way of death. It is the story of the man who had two sons, better known as the story of the prodigal son.

> There was a man who had two sons; and the younger of them said to his father, "Father, give me the share of the property that falls to me." And he divided his living between them. Not many days later, the younger son gathered all that he had and took his journey into a far country, and there he squandered his property in loose living. And when he had spent everything, a great famine arose in that country, and he began to be in want. So he went and joined himself to one of the citizens of that country, who sent him into his fields

> to feed swine. And he would gladly have fed on the pods that the swine ate, and no one gave him anything. But when he came to himself he said, "How many of my father's hired servants have bread enough and to spare, but I perish here with hunger! I will arise and go to my father, and I will say to him, 'Father, I have sinned against heaven and before you; I am no longer worthy to be called your son; treat me as one of your hired servants.'
>
> And he arose and came to his father. But while he was yet at a distance, his father saw him and had compassion, and ran and embraced him and kissed him. And the son said to him, "Father, I have sinned against heaven and before you; I am no longer worthy to be called your son." But the father said to his servants, "Bring the best robe, and put it on him; and put a ring on his hand and shoes on his feet; and bring the fatted calf and kill it, and let us eat and make merry; for this my son was dead, and is alive again; he was lost and is found." And they began to make merry. (Luke 15:11–24)

The story continues with a vignette involving the other brother who confronts the father in a jealous rage, questioning why the father would be so gracious to this son who had wasted his share of the family fortune, especially when he, himself, had served the father so faithfully 'lo these many years' and had not even a goat to feast on with *his* friends. The other side of staying home and working for father is the freedom of travel, independence, and the self indulgence which anonymity can encourage. The other side of being rich enough to throw money away is being so penniless and hungry that even what the pigs are eating begins to look good. The other side of reckless abandon in the anonymity afforded by "a far country" is coming to yourself, waking up to who you really are, regaining your true identity. The other side of running away from home is running toward it, an action which, as in our story, must be preceded by a change deep in consciousness. The desire to escape is replaced by the desire to return. It is seeing the light in the midst of darkness. It is being first dead to the truth of the power of love freely given and then alive to realization of that truth. It is being lost and then found.

Theologically, this is a story which celebrates the magnetic power of love and forgiveness, and lets the reader know that the story teller believes the kingdom where those qualities exist is the side which always manifests in the long run. In the words of the prologue to the Gospel of John, "The light shines on in the dark, and the darkness has never quenched it," (John 1:5). The darkness is there, it is the back side of light, but in a universe whose basic nature is Light, darkness is a transitory phenomenon. The prodigal, when he had come to himself, lived out the injunction in Ephesians (a call to go from back to front): ". . . leaving your former way of life, you must lay aside that old human nature which, deluded by its lusts, is sinking towards death. You must be made new in mind and spirit, and put on the new nature of God's creating, which shows itself in the just and devout life called for by the truth," (Ephesians 3:22–24).

The order of the universe, the will of God, the divine economy, the dynamic interplay of the manifestation of the seven principles, the law of the Lord: all these are descriptions of the ultimate reality. This reality becomes our dominant mode of understanding and the ground for our behavior again and again in life as we turn from error to truth, from darkness to light, from back to front until, finally, it is the only side in which we invest the energy of our attention and, in so doing, to which we give life. This is not to say that the darkness is not there, that there are no back sides to the fronts. This is to say that we can recognize the negatives the way we recognize people who walk into a room while we are engrossed in reading: by acknowledging their presence and then getting back to what we are doing, rather than by turning our attention to them and engaging them in conversation which then becomes what we are doing.

The poor in spirit are blessed precisely because they have richness of the things of the spirit to which to look forward. The other side of emptiness is fullness. There is hope for the hopeless. The song of Mary, recorded in Luke as Mary's response to the annunciation, is a litany of backs and fronts. This scripture passage is used regularly in worship in churches which retain the fullest liturgical tradition. It is found in Luke 1:46–55 and describes the overturning of things as they existed at the dawn of the coming of the Kingdom of God, that state of consciousness where the first are last and the last first. Mary, the lowly handmaiden, is described as henceforth being called blessed by all generations; that typically tight group of the proud are "scattered"; the mighty have been dethroned, and the humble and meek exalted; the hungry have been filled with good things, and the rich sent away empty.

The early believers who deemed such a statement worth preserving as a part of the gospel record did so because their whole faith was centered around the recognition of the necessary existence of fronts and backs, a pair of which lay at the heart of the good news—death and life. They believed that their master demonstrated that neither death nor life can stand alone, that the living will die and the dying will live. Since this universal truth, described by the principles of fronts and backs seems so obvious, one wonders why the particular Christian application of it—death and resurrection— has been such a stumbling block to those outside that faith.

The Sermon on The Mount, found in the fifth chapter of Matthew and cast by Luke as The Sermon on the Plain in the sixth chapter of that gospel, is a catalogue of the teachings of Jesus on the inevitability of change from back to front and the hope implicit in that change. It is a description of life in the Kingdom of God, that inner and outer place where the lawful appropriateness of the manifestation of the order of the universe is understood and celebrated as God's Will.

The following quotation sums up the necessity of complementary and proportional fronts and backs in order for there to be any manifestation at all. Therefore, it also plumbs the depths of what it means to be human. It is by Fiona MacLeod, the *nom de plume* of William Sharpe, from his book, *Isle of Dreams*.

How can one understand the joy that is so near to sorrow, the sorrow that like a wave of the sea can break in a moment into light and beauty?

I have heard often in effect, "This is no deep heart that in one hour weeps, and in the next laughs." but I know a deeper heart that in one hour weeps and in the next laughs, so deep that light dies away within it, and silence and the beginning and the end are one: the heart of the sea. And there is another heart that is deep and weeps one hour and in the next laughs: the heart of night: where oblivion smiles and it is day, sighs, and the darkness comes. And there is another heart that is deep and weeps in one hour and in the next laughs: the soul of man: where tears and laughter are the fans that blow the rose-white flame of life.[2]

---

[1] Chesterton, *Francis of Assisi,* pp. 96, 97.
[2] MacLeod, *The Isle of Dreams,* p. 123.

Chapter 6

What has a Beginning has an End

"Heaven and earth will pass away;
my words will never pass away."
(Mark 13 : 31a)

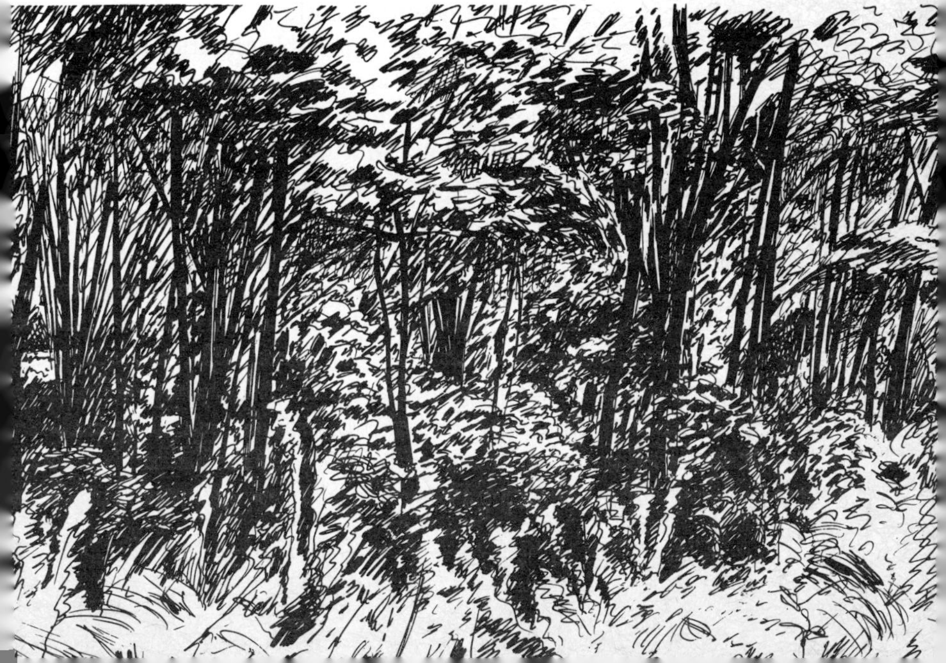

THERE ARE TWO PHRASES I HEARD AS A CHILD which I remember as being particularly frustrating. One was the often heard response to a request: "We'll see." The other was an explanation of why whatever enjoyable behavior had to stop, usually because it was time to leave, go to bed, or meet some other adult scheduling requirement: "All good things must come to an end." I did not want the thing being engaged in to come to an end whether it was good, bad, or somewhere in between, and yet, all those good things *did* come to an end. They had begun and so they ended. The last of the seven principles is another way of saying the same thing, and it could be argued, from the Christian viewpoint, that in a universe produced by a creator who "saw everything that he had made, and behold, it was very good," (Genesis 1:31a) the childhood version is more accurate theologically. The seventh principle advises us that all good things, everything which has a beginning, must one day cease to be.

There are creation and destruction stories in every culture. Hinduism even personalizes the forces of creation and destruction in Shiva and Kali who are married to each other as "beginning" is to "end" in the statement of the seventh principle. The Bible offers two stories of the creation of the world in the first and second chapters of Genesis, and many possible scenarios for the world's destruction, some of which are in direct contradiction. Modern science has offered the big bang theory of creation and the second law of thermodynamics which states, essentially, that all of creation is descending into chaos—the state of the universe which the first chapter of Genesis describes as existing before creation. We are participants in a multi-billion-year old drama of beginnings and endings, perceiving the very scene in which we find ourselves with senses which are, themselves, moving toward their end.

When examining theories of the creation of the universe advanced by western science one cannot help but be struck by how fantastic they seem. These theories are, at first blush, no less fantastic than the Genesis story which is accepted as literal fact by those within the ranks of Christendom who consider the Bible to be absolutely true, scientifically, and historically, as written. Let us look at one small part of science's attempt to explain how it all began: the problem of why matter and anti-matter did not simply annihilate each other, resulting in a universe which would have lasted a billionth of a second at the moment of the "big bang."

As has been said, all the universal principles apply all the time. In considering our sub-problem we see all of our principles in operation. First there exists an undifferentiated One; no thing has been created. At the moment of creation two things arise, a front and a back, proportional and complementary. Science calls these two things matter and anti-matter. Remember, we said that when anything arises it comes in two parts or it does not exist at all. Immediately, these various, non-identical, forms of matter and their corresponding anti-matter begin to change. Because of the nature of their complementarity their particular form of change is that they cancel each other out, and with mutual annihilation is released the energy which it took to create them. The problem is: if this is true, why are we here? The answer which science gives us is wonderfully creative, quasi-theological, and definitely no more or less believable than Genesis 1.

Some astrophysicists have said when matter and antimatter managed to escape each other's clutches, (defy the fronts and backs principles) and retreat to enormous regions composed of only one type. This means that whole galaxies could be composed of anti-matter. The only problem with this explanation is that no theorist has been able to come up with a way for this separation to have occured. Another minor suspension of the rules (a supernatural event?) has been suggested by the big bang people, so minor that it really does not do terrible violence to the rules, but it does allow for why we really *are* here after all. This theory is an outgrowth of the search for scientific proof that everything is a differentiation of one infinity, although science calls this the search for a unified field theory. This theory would treat the four scientifically recognized forces of nature—gravitational, electromagnetic, weak nuclear, and strong nuclear—as different expressions of the same basic interaction. The theory runs, roughly, as follows: at a temperature of a billion billion billion degrees, such as would have existed during the first billion-billion-billionth of a second at the big bang moment, for every billion anti-protons created there could have been a billion and one protons produced. So, too, other atomic particles which we would consider as being matter would have outnumbered their complementary opposites, anti-matter. One has to presume that, if we lived in an anti-matter galaxy, it would seem like matter to us, and what we now consider to be matter would be perceived as anti-matter. Although this one part per billion of leftover matter seems like an inconceivably small amount of extra matter, when dealing with astronomical proportions it would allow for the existence of the universe as we know it—galaxies, suns, and planets. This means that our local universe is a fluke occurence composed of warmed up leftovers; warmed by the enormous heat created by the mutual annihilation of matter and anti-matter. In fact, when the heat remaining from the big bang is measured the results are impressive in their power to support this theory.

To the believer whose cosmology finds its roots in the language and imagery of the Bible, the question of what happened in the beginning is answered in the first verse of the first chapter of that book, "In the beginning God created the heavens and the earth." If that believer is a fundamentalist, the succeeding verses of the first chapter of Genesis advise about details of the creation process. If the believer understands that the Genesis creation story tells the universal truth that God created the heavens and the earth (that creation proceeds from one infinity) in what manner we are still discovering, then the story is viewed as a myth. A myth is a story which tells a universal truth but whose trappings may not, themselves, be universally true. The author of Genesis 1 used the current wisdom of his day to describe the creation process, a description which follows the sequence of the theory elaborated by Darwin to a remarkable degree. The writer recalled oral traditions, legends, and what could be called the "science" of the day, weaving all this into the details of the Genesis story to describe fully the universal truth—God created the heavens and the earth. The Genesis narrative certainly appeals to the poetic wonder implicit in human nature in reporting God as saying, "Let there be light," rather than "Let there be left overs," but current wisdom could report the latter as the initial creative command.

The greatest difficulty in any discussion of things Biblical is the Bible's use of anthropomorphic images in describing the deity—making God in our image. This use is due to the natural desire of Biblical writers to ascribe to God the attributes of the most evolved beings known to them. Therefore, those attributes are human. The difficulty is that human beings are *not* infinite, not outside of time and space while walking the earth. Although there are aspects of the human condition such as spirit and love which participate in the infinite, when God is described as giving commands, being angry, having time and space limitations, seated on a throne ruling like a middle eastern king, sooner or later such a description breaks down under the weight of the limitations it imposes. We must not fault the Biblical writers for describing the deity in their ancient manner, but we *do* bear some responsibility to translate such limiting descriptions into more comfortable terminology rather than being so put off by the necessity of having to do so that we turn our backs on the truths being described. This is not an easy task, however, and its attempt has spawned many heretics especially as measured by those who are attached to the concrete images of the grandfatherly figure "up there." Paul Tillich's "ground of our being" is such an attempt which modern theology finds acceptable. Yet there are those who would rather it had been "ground of our meeting," since it is in relationships that the infinite breaks in on the human condition most forcefully. The spiritualist churches refer to God as "infinite intelligence" which seems somewhat restrictive. Surely he is infinite everything else as well. In the Judo-Christian tradition the infinite is given gender, and today's theological scene is littered with the remains of battle being done by those who would prefer inclusive language and those who insist that the traditional masculine designation does no violence to the intention of inclusiveness. In macrobiotic literature the deity is referred to as "one infinity," and, although this is accurate it certainly lacks the personal quality of the Christian use of "Father." Actually "Daddy" would be a more accurate translation of "Abba." But, then, is the creator not "Mother" too? So there are those, especially from the "New Thought Movement" of the latter 19th century, who refer to "Father-Mother God." The central point of all this is a reminder that the deity is not a being having qualities, but *is those qualities.* The American mystic, Joel Goldsmith, has said, "All that can be said about God is that he is, and he is 'is-ing.'" Toward the end of the time when New Testament writings were produced there was profound Greek influence on the theology of the early Church and the writer of the Gospel of John reflects that unusual abstractive quality in referring to God as "light" (1 John 1:5) and "love" (1 John 4:9). Of particular interest to the subject of this chapter is John The Divine's report that the risen Christ, the deity manifest, refers to himself as "The Alpha and the Omega, the beginning and the end" no less than four times in The Book of Revelation, (1:8, 1:11, 21:6, 22:13). Thus, what has a beginning has an end, and both beginning and end, as well as what comes between them, are where the divine may be encountered: in creation, existence, and destruction, in the regular, the ordinary, the universal occurrences which comprise our daily lives.

"God said," recurs in Genesis 1, on the occasion of each act of creation. It is by the power of God's word that things are called into being: "By the word of the Lord the heavens were made," (Psalm 33:6). The natural order obeys the word which created them: ". . . fire and hail, snow and frost, stormy wind fulfilling his command," (Psalm 148:8). It is the "word of the Lord" which communicates divine will to the prophets of the Old Testament. Word is a vehicle for showing forth the one whom Paul describes as dwelling "in unapproachable light," (1 Timothy 6:16). During the intertestamental period the *logos* or "word" attained a personal quality and became more explicitly viewed as an intermediary: "Thy all powerful word leaped from heaven, from the royal throne, into the midst of the land that was doomed, a stern warrior carrying the sharp sword of thy authentic command," (Wisdom of Solomon 18:15). As the understanding of the power and function of the "Word" evolved, the way was paved for its use in the New Testament. "The Word" is used to describe the incarnation of the intermediary (1 John 2:1) as well as the incarnation of divinity and humanity, (Mark 1:1, 1:11, and occasions when Jesus refers to himself as 'The Son of Man'). The Gospel of John goes even further and establishes the "Word" as equal to the creator. In the powerful theology of John's prologue to that book:

> When all things began, the Word already was. The Word dwelt with God, and what God was the Word was. The Word, then, was with God at the beginning, and through him all things came to be; no single thing was created without him. All that came to be was alive with his life, and that life was the light of men. The light shines on in the dark and the darkness has never quenched it. (1 John : 1–5)

The Word, which the Wisdom quote described as having "leaped from heaven," is portrayed by John as back on the throne, and John The Divine hears this word as "Alpha and Omega, the beginning and the end," referred to above. We find a continuity of development here resulting in the equating of the "Word" spoken by God with creative and redemptive power, a power made flesh in the person of Jesus. Therefore, for the Christian, the act of creation is inextricable not only from faith in God the father, but from the person of the Christ described by the Nicene Creed as the One "through whom all things were made."

Appearing as it does in the last and most recently written book in the Bible, the "Alpha and Omega" formula demonstrates the ultimate theological refinement of identifying the Christ with both the beginning and the end. However, in some of the earliest New Testament writings we find very specific descriptions of how the risen Christ will intervene at the end time. This end time, when the intervention will take place, is a continuation of the Old Testament understanding that the cosmos will undergo a decisive, divine act which will usher in a new age. That moment is called "The Day of The Lord" in the Old Testament, and the coming of "The Kingdom of God" in the New Testament. Early Christianity gave this moment the name, "The Second Coming of Christ."

The evolution of concepts regarding the nature of the end time are recorded over a period of nearly one thousand years in biblical writing, and the change which occurred over that many years is obvious. The earliest notions of the coming of the Day of The Lord find their roots in the accounts of creation, since divine intervention in the end time implies belief in divine activity at the beginning. Old Testament eschatology (the study of the end time) is one more application of the biblical belief in the divinity at work in history. In the case of the end time the intervention is understood to mean the end of history as we know it. There is no anticipation that the end will be total annihilation, or a return to the chaos which existed as the precursor of creation. The end is understood, rather, as a refinement of present conditions, not without some catastrophic acts, which will result in the realization of God's rule, known as the coming of his kingdom. It will be a theocracy, a new dispensation, a higher turn of the spiral, qualitatively different from a simple cyclical return to a former point on a circle.

Behind the belief in the coming era, however, *does* lie an echo of the pagan celebration of yearly cycles of nature which renew the earth through annual floods, the expectation of spring run-offs, and the return of the planting season with the new life which comes with the death of the seed. Since, as in all history, whatever occurs is a part of the divine economy and part of "the Will of God," there is implicit hope even in the midst of graphic descriptions of the destruction which the last day will bring.

Nowhere in the Old Testament is that description filled with more violent imagery than in the Book of The Prophet Zephaniah who for this reason has been called the prophet of The Day of The Lord. Zephaniah's descriptions combine cosmic and political terrors, events of wars and natural catastrophes.

> The great day of the Lord is near, near and hastening fast; the sound of the day of the Lord is bitter, the mighty man cries aloud there. A day of wrath is that day, a day of distress and anguish, a day of ruin and devastation, a day of darkness and gloom, a day of clouds and thick darkness, a day of trumpet blast and battle cry against the fortified cities and against the lofty battlements. (Zephaniah 1: 14–16)

How did such fantastic imagery evolve as a description of the end time? It came out of the need of the prophets to point out to an errant and faithless people the foolishness of their ways and the penalty for such apostasy. The oldest passage mentioning the day of the Lord occurs in Amos 5: 18–20:

> Woe to you who desire the day of the Lord! Why would you have the day of the Lord? It is darkness and not light; is not the day of the Lord darkness and not light and gloom with no brightness in it?

It was this prophet who told the people of Israel that God would carry out the divine plan through surrounding enemy nations thus extending the "concern" of the deity for nations other than the chosen people. Amos was warning his hearers that the day of the Lord would be ushered in through, among other things, political defeat. These do not sound like implicitly hopeful words! The implicit hope is found in a parallel understanding which, like the day of the Lord, already existed in the people's theological vocabulary before being enunciated by their prophets. This concept is that of the faithful remnant who will be saved from destruction on the "Day." This salvation will come because of their faithfulness, the right use of their place in the divine economy, and, in Old Testament terms, because of their abiding by the Law of the Lord.

> Hate evil and love good, and establish justice in the gate; it may be that the Lord the God of hosts, will be gracious to the remnant of Joseph. (Amos 5: 15)

> In that day I will raise up the booth of David that is fallen and repair its breaches, and raise up its ruins, and rebuild it as in the days of old. (Amos 9: 11)

> "I will restore the fortunes of my people Israel, and they shall rebuild the ruined cities and inhabit them; they shall plant vineyards and drink their wine, and they shall make gardens and eat their fruit. I will plant them upon the land and they shall never again be plucked up out of the land which I have given them," says the Lord your God. (Amos 9: 14–15)

In later Old Testament writings also appears the expectation that the Day would be ushered in by two figures, one a forerunner and preparer of the way for the other personage, the Messiah or anointed one.[1] Although understood to be addressed to the political situation of his time, namely the Syrian-Ephraimitic War (734-733 B.C.), the messianic expectation described by Isaiah is a passage often used in connection with Christmas celebrations:

> For to us a child is born, to us a son is given; and the government will be upon his shoulder, and his name will be called "Wonderful, Counselor, Mighty God, Everlasting Father, Prince of Peace." Of the increase of his government and of peace there will be no end, upon the throne of David, and over his kingdom, to establish it, and to uphold it with justice and with righteousness from this time forth for ever-

> more. The zeal of the Lord of hosts will do this. (Isaiah 9:6, 7)

Early Christians believed that Jesus was that anointed one, the Messiah or Christ, and therefore looked to the scriptures predicting the return of Elijah (as the forerunner) and the coming of the Messiah to be a prophecy about John the Baptizer and Jesus. This identification was enhanced by the use in the Greek Old Testament of the word "Lord where in the Hebrew God was called Yahweh. Thus the day of Yahweh became the day of the Lord, a name Christians used to address Jesus. Paul even uses the term "The day of the Lord Jesus," in 1 Corinthians 5:5, and identifies the second coming with "the day of the Lord" in 2 Thessalonians 2:1, 2. Paul's belief in the immanent return of Jesus so colors his writings that they often cannot be understood without realizing that fact. He even states in I Thessalonians that some who hear his words read will be alive when Jesus returns, and he goes on to describe the manner in which the return will be effected:

> For this we declare to you by the word of the Lord, that we who are alive, who are left until the coming of the Lord, shall not precede those who have fallen asleep. For the Lord himself will descend from heaven with a cry of command, with the archangel's call, and with the sound of the trumpet of God. And the dead in Christ will rise first; then we who are alive, who are left, shall be caught up together with them in the clouds to meet the Lord in the air; and so we shall always be with the Lord. Therefore comfort one another with these words. (1 Thessalonians 4:15–18)

Paul was wrong if we are to take his words literally, and it certainly seems to be how those words were intended. Apocalypticism, belief in the immanence of the end time, was rampant in the centuries immediately preceding Jesus facilitating the identity of Jesus with the Messiah by his disciples. In the years following the resurrection there had to be some adjustment in eschatalogy since the end of the physical world did not happen with Jesus' ministry and the sinful were still in their midst! Sinners had not been eradicated as predicted in the Old Testament as part of the Messianic plan. He must have to return to complete the plan at "the end of the age," (Matthew 28:20).

That expectation not only colors Paul's writings, it is also reflected in the Gospels and other New Testament letters. Accounts vary as details are described by different writers, but the persistence of apocalyptic expectations carries through the New Testament period and through the life of the church to the present day. Throughout the history of the Church serious and devout believers have boarded up their homes and shops and gathered to wait for the moment. Each time they have had to return to the life they thought they were leaving as the second coming failed to materialize according to their expectations. There are those today within fundamentalist Christianity who can point to the Book of Revelation, also known as the Apocalypse of St. John The Divine, and find predictions of the atomic tests conducted in the Anawetok Atoll, the army of The Soviet Union, identification of cities in Siberia, and the exact place where the first nuclear blast will occur.

When the world situation is perceived to be difficult, aplocalypticism blooms with new zeal, and the present time has engendered just such activity. By no one's expectation could the coming of the eschaton be seen as "the easy way out." Wherever apocalypticism arises it is accompanied by expectations of phenomenal difficulty as well as hope for a surviving remnant, even if that survival is in matter finer than that of the physical world. The case was made by Jerome Canty for the return of Quetzelcoatl as Cortez, in his execllent book, *Sounding The Sacred Conch.* Likewise, a case could well be made for the second coming of the Christ as the purging fire of nuclear holocaust. The destruction of, at least, the planet is well within humanity's grasp. If predictions of the date of the "return" have been wrong then it is not too far fetched to assume that the nature of the return may also be wrongly predicted. Since the second coming did not come when Paul and other New Testament writers expected, nor has it come when any number of adventist groups packed up to await it, nor has the physical world yet been destroyed as often predicted by secular apocalypticists, perhaps the expectation of physical cataclysm and establishment of an outer theocracy is in error. The belief in a future "coming" of the Messiah is firmly part of the Christian and Jewish faiths. Christianity believes that he has come and will return. Judaism holds that he has not yet come. All this pertains to the future, but what about the present?

The one whom Christians believe to be the Messiah taught that the Kingdom of God was not just a future event but a present reality. He declared that he was ushering in the end time by his activity (Mark 1:15), and that the Kingdom could be found within believers. (Luke 17:21) There is, then, more than an intimation in Jesus' teaching that the end time has already come. The years following the resurrection did *not* see the arrival of events as they had been predicted in the law and the prophets. Rome was not overthrown and the monarchy established with its center at Jerusalem. A second coming therefore must be necessary to bring this to pass. The early phase of the preaching of the church as recorded in Paul's epistles and the early gospels shows a strong final eschatology. This can be seen in Acts 3:21 and 1 Corinthians 15:23–28. However, the original teaching of Jesus seems to have been recovered by the time the Gospel of John was written, toward the end of the first century. Perhaps it was recognized that much of what had been predicted in the Old Testament had come to pass as an internal, personal reality rather than as a political occurrence. Jesus' words, "my kingdom is not of this world," (John 18:36) reflect this evolution of understanding. The eschaton had been realized. The kingdom had come. We are participating in the life of the eternal One *now*: "The one who hears my word and has faith in Him who sent me possesses eternal life . . . he has passed from death to life." (John 5:24)

The Johanine Christian[2] did not think that one needs to

> wait until the second coming to see God: whoever has seen Jesus has seen the Father, as Jesus said, "From now on you do know him and have seen him." (John 14:7–10)[3]

The implications of always being in the end time are nothing short of astounding to a world view which sees beginnings and endings as points at each end of a straight line continuum. Jesus' teaching of "realized eschatology," as it is known in theology, also casts an interesting light on the principle that what has a beginning has an end. No longer can we see the principle simply as describing a linear process of starts and finishes but as applying to the birth and death of each moment as well. A myriad of beginnings and endings comprise the world as we perceive it. This principle, then, partakes of principle two, that everything changes. All beginnings are moving toward their end by processes which themselves are beginning and ending.

It is no wonder that in both Christian theology and macrobiotic philosophy the goal of union with the unchanging and eternal is seen as the ultimate state. In both understandings the sublime stability of that ultimate state is accessible here and now through realization of the kingdom of God. This realization is effected in Christian theology by knowledge of the Truth which makes one free. Such knowledge is not a simple cognitive exercise but an experiential knowing in one's heart through faith in the One described by the writer of John as "full of grace and truth," (John 1:14).

George Ohsawa defines the kingdom of God as the state entered through understanding the laws of the Order of the Universe: the seven universal principles and the Laws of Change.

> The truth of the Order of the Universe as Jesus Christ says, confirms that with this order one can achieve everything without the need for any instruments: "Seek truth and truth will liberate you," (John 8:32). And again: "So, above all, look for the kingdom and the justice of God and all the rest will be given to you in addition," (Matthew 6:33).

> The kingdom of God can be nothing else than the absolute-eternal-infinite and its tangible justice, the Order of the Universe, which lead and govern everything. When one has this order well in hand one can build on the antagonistic complementarity.[4]

The reign of God, or the coming of the kingdon, as a personal event rather than an historical/political one has ample biblical justification. Jesus' teachings about the kingdom of heaven in what biblical scholars call "the parables of the kingdom" describe a state of consciousness, a mode of behavior, a way of viewing the world of phenomena. In particular, Luke records Jesus as saying, "The kingdom of God is not coming with signs to be observed; nor will they say, "Lo, here it is!" or "There!" for behold, the kingdom of God is in the midst of you,"[5] (Luke 17:20b–21). Paul's teachings stress the union of the believer with the risen Christ and the human spirit with the Spirit of God the Father prompting the cry, "Abba, Father," (Romans 8:15). He even states that the believer has "the mind of Christ,"[6] (1 Corinthians 2:16). When the Messiah comes, the coming will be experienced in one's deepest being since the Messiah is the incarnation of the One "in whom we live and move and have our being," (Acts 17:28).

> The New Testament scholar, James Breech, observes: Jesus states quite clearly that the kingdom of which he speaks is not a coming kingdom, a future kingdom, for it is already in the midst of his listeners. As soon as the kingdom is spoken of as a present reality, its character is changed. Obviously, the set of conceptions which associates the kingdom with a factual transformation or ending of the world is abrogated. Neither God, nor his Messiah, nor his angels, nor any other transcendental beings have intervened from a mythological heaven. . . .[7]

Michio Kushi reflects this same understanding with a remarkably similar sentiment. The following statement was made by him in answer to the question, "When the Messiah comes, is our salvation achieved from this misery?"

> The Messiah never comes under the name of "Messiah." The Messiah is not a person who comes to some place at some time. When you talk about salvation, you are forgetting this infinite universe and its endless order, within which you are born and which is always in front of you. The awareness that you are a manifestation of this infinite universe is the true Messiah, and when you know yourself, you save yourself, finding that you are within the endless happiness of life.[8]

Perhaps the reason that realized eschatology is not found more obviously in popular Christian teaching is because the futuristic expectation of the coming kingdom relieves one from manifesting the Christ consciousness in the present moment. Realized eschatology means real responsiblity without appeal to an "I'm only human" excuse. It would be difficult to beg off one's shortcomings with the words, "I'm only the temple of the Holy Spirit with the mind of Christ."

The Right Reverend Paul Moore, Jr., Episcopal Bishop of New York, even sees the dominance of traditional apocalypticism in present day fundamentalism as a lack of hope:

> Already the need for primitive symbolism is seen in the attraction of the modern Fundamentalists. It may be a death wish that draws the followers of the Moral Majority toward the literal interpretation of Armageddon as a cosmic Jonestown. It may be a longing for the thunder of Yahweh, so long absent from American middle-class Protestantism, or it may be a desperate abandonment of hope for this created world.[9]

Realized eschatology is made real through awareness, the subject matter of Chapter 11. However, whether the end time is viewed as a future event or as a present reality by the Christian believer there is no separating it from the Christ "through whom all things were made"[10] and who will come again (in realized eschatology that coming occurs again, again, and again) at the end time. His is, indeed, an Alpha and Omega presence a part from whom nothing exists, present at the beginning and the end. In fact, whatever presence is recognized as being there at both the beginning and the end by any religion is that same presence, the incarnation of the infinite One.

One of the most startling end times to behold is that of the end of the life of the physical body. As natural an event as it is there is still an air of tremendous mystery that consciousness within the physical frame should suddenly exist only outside the body. A person is in our midst at one moment and the next they are gone. Although it is true that "in the midst of life we are in death," we are still so surprised by its coming that the vast majority of bereaved follow a series of stages of grief which begins as shock and denial. It is, as Paul says, "the last enemy to be overcome," (1 Corinthians 15:26) not that it is to be avoided through eternal life of the body but that understanding and dealing with it is the most difficult of those isues faced within the human condition. Religions worldwide postulate paradises, heavens, and glorified states of being detailed as afterlife rewards to put the death of the body in a more comfortable context. There is no doubt in my heart and mind that the human consciousness continues after death and that death is simply the door to another life. But when it comes unexpectedly to someone we love no philosophy on earth can obviate the heart-rending grief process. Death is a great advisor and, as a universal, a great leveler. It has happened to all in the past and will happen to all in the future whether they dwell in the public eye or in obscurity. "Your life, what is it? You are no more than a mist, seen for a little while then dispersing," (James 4:14).

Those who have been declared clinically dead and then revived report that they are no longer afraid of death. They have passed through it and, in some cases, found their experiences "on the other side" very attractive. Still, the Grim Reaper is pictured as stalking us and waiting until "our time is up." To the wise the presence of death gives renewed meaning to each day of life as a stimulus for gratitude and an encouragement to make the best use of our time. Death's unavoidability in its universality makes it fearful psychologically. We would rather not think about it. Running counter to the instinct to survive, death is also fearful at a very deep level of being. The following story is a classic and, in dramatic imagery, captures both the fear and the unavoidability of the end of life in the body.

> Once a wealthy merchant of Baghdad sent a beloved servant to the marketplace to purchase provisions. Within minutes the servant had returned and was pounding at the door shaking and covered with perspiration. "While I was in the marketplace I met Death and he threatened me with his fists," the servant sobbed, "I must borrow your fastest horse and make for far off Samara immediately. Death will never find me there!" Permission was granted and the servant galloped off for the distant city.
>
> The more the merchant thought about the state of his poor servant the angrier he became. At last he could contain himself no longer and went to the marketplace. He found Death in the crowd and accosted him with, "Why did you threaten my servant with your fists when you met him here earlier? He is a loyal and faithful soul and not deserving of such treatment!"
>
> Death replied, "I did not threaten him! My fists were raised suddenly in a gesture of surprise. I was shocked to see him here in Babhdad, for I have an appointment with him tonight in far off Samara."

Since the ongoing life of the human spirit is a universal truth there are descriptions of the nature of this life in every culture. These descriptions may vary in detail from the highly specific images of the progression of the spirit through bardo levels in Northern Buddhism to Christian burial prayers describing the deceased as going "from strength to strength in the life of perfect service." What these traditions recognize is that death is the end of the body and not annihilation of the total being. There is no ultimate separation in this world which has proceeded from the infinite One, and there is no way to separate the creation from the creator. The hope implicit in our first principle of the infinite universe is realized in the last principle when applied to the last thing we will do in this world of physical phenomena. Just as God could ask Job where he was when the foundation of the earth was laid (Job 38: 4), so, too, there is a state of being which is appropriate to the time when that which is of the earth is destroyed. The latter "place" is the same as the former: ". . . at home with the Lord," (2 Corinthians 5: 8).

> For I am convinced that there is nothing in death or life, in the realm of spirits or superhuman powers, in the world as it is or in the world as it shall be, in the forces of the universe, in heights or depths—nothing in all creation that can separate us from the love of God in Christ Jesus our Lord. (Romans 8: 38, 39)

The stairs which Jacob saw leading from earth to heaven (Genesis 28: 12) are a spiral staircase. They lead from the One down into the many. All have descended those stairs at the beginning of life, and all will ascend them again when their life in the realm of change has come to its end. In truth, we are descending and ascending every step of those stairs simultaneously. If we will but remember from whence we came the awareness of where we are going brings joy to the journey—infinite joy.

---

[1] see Malachi 4:5.

[2] Those who followed the school of thought represented by the writer of the Gospel and Epistles of John.

[3] Brown, *The Community of The Beloved Disciple*, p. 51.
[4] From *The Book of Judo, Macromuse*, Issue 14.
[5] The Greek word translated "midst" can also mean "within."
[6] The Greek word translated "mind" has a broader meaning and might be translated "character." It encompasses more than mental qualities.
[7] Breech, *The Silence of Jesus*, p. 36.
[8] Kushi, *The Book of Macrobiotics*, p. 96.
[9] *The Witness*, Vol. 68, Number 1, "Meditation for a Nuclear Age," The Rt. Rev. Paul Moore, Jr., p. 8.
[10] The Nicene Creed.

PART II

The Heart of Macrobiotics and Christianity

Chapter 7

Yin and Yang

"In the beginning God created the heavens and the earth." (Genesis 1 : 1)

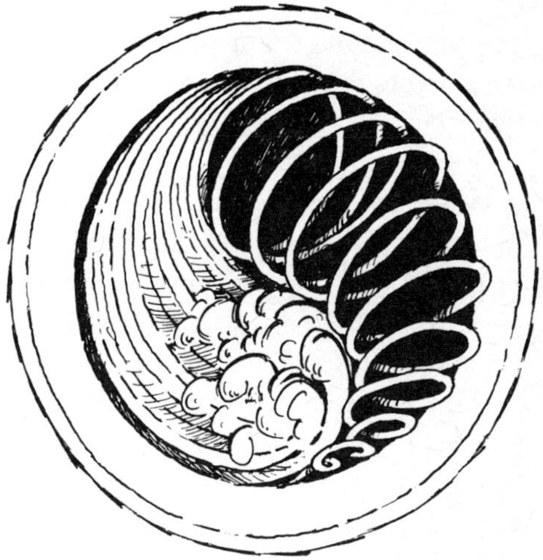

THERE IS NO MENTION OF YIN AND YANG in the Seven Universal Principles of the Infinite Universe. This startling fact should advise us of the true universality of the principles. They may be interpreted in verbal categories to which yin and yang are foreign. However, macrobiotic literature abounds with descriptions of the manifestation of these two tendencies in disease, food, lifestyle, physiognomy, cosmology, and a multitude of other categories. Although the terms yin and yang are oriental in origin, using those words to describe the universal occurrence of complementary tendencies in creating any manifestation has been appreciated in the West. It would be possible to evolve a totally Western interpretation of the principles without the use of yin and yang, but adopting the use of these two words for expansive and contractive tendencies, as they are used in macrobiotic philosophy, is not only easier but desirable. Words with similar meaning in the English language usually carry some connotative value as in "plus and minus," "positive and negative," "up and down," "light and dark," "hot and cold," "contraction and expansion." There is a purity inherent in words free from previous associations. They may be used with good result in building new understandings. For most Westerners one of the most unfamiliar concepts found in macrobiotic philosophy is the use of yin and yang.

Yin and yang are not entities. They are tendencies. There is no such thing as a yin or a yang nor can one tendency exist without the other. These words simply describe the processes of fluctuation which have been observed throughout the centuries, designations for what has been observed by many philosophers and scientists in cultures throughout the world. In macrobiotics the terms refer to the tendency to expansion and contraction or those states reflecting the dominance of one tendency over another. When David slew Goliath he used a balancing of these tendencies to keep his sling whirling before sending the stone on its way. As he whirled the sling around his head the expansive centrifugal force kept the stone at the limit of the cords which held the pouch. The cords communicated the contractive centripetal force being applied to the cords by David's hand preventing the whole device from flying out of his grasp.

On a cosmic scale this same application keeps planets on their courses, galaxies from flying apart or collapsing in upon themselves, creating a balancing act of truly astronomic proportions:

> There is much competition to be found in nature, between the balance and interplay of different forces, for instance. A star is a battleground of opposing forces. Gravity, which tries to crush the star, struggles against the forces of thermal pressure and electromagnetic radiation which try to explode it—forces which in turn are generated by the release of energy due to nuclear interactions. And all across the universe the struggle goes on. However, if the forces were not more or less equally matched, all physical systems would be overwhelmed by one or the other, and activity would cease. The universe is complex and interesting precisely because these battles continue over the aeons.[1]

Compared with our tiny size the tendency toward balance sometimes takes on aspects of "battle" and "struggle" when observed at the galactic level, but according to the principles of the infinite universe we know that this is no battle or struggle. The universe is not at war with itself. All antagonisms are complementary.

"Yin" and "yang" are the designations used by ancient Chinese philosophers and, thus, today in the orient in general. The order of the universe was seen by Heraclitus as a flickering fire, "kindling in measures and going out in measures." Empedocles saw the ebb and flow of primal forces as "love" and "hate." The Aztec culture used categories of "hot" and "cold" in their medical theory. Modern philosophers and scientists have coined their own terms. Saint-Simon used "organic" and "critical"; Herbert Spencer saw a series of "integrations" and "differentiations" as constituting cosmic movements. Hegel viewed all of human history as spirallic, moving from unity to a phase of disunity then to reintegration on a higher turn of that spiral. Arthur Koestler, in his book *Janus,* has coined the word "holons" for parts of systems, with each "holon" being composed of the two tendencies of "integration" and "self assertion." Arnold Toynbee used "challenge" and "response" to give meaning to the great movements of history, deciding that "yin" and "yang" are appropriate and helpful even to a Western mind:

> Of the various symbols in which different observers in different societies have expressed the alternation between a static condition and a dynamic activity in the rhythm of the Universe, Yin and Yang are the most apt, because they convey the measure of the rhythm directly and not through some metaphor derived from psychology or mechanics or mathematics.[2]

The words "yin" and "yang" do not occur, as such, within the Judeo-Christian tradition, but the tendencies designated appear often in biblical writing, sometimes explicitly. The very first verse of Genesis recognizes these two qualities in the first act of creation, quantifying them with the words, "In the beginning God created the heavens and the earth." If we look at the yin and yang qualities of heaven and earth we begin to understand why, although the basic yin/yang theory is simple, its practical application can become complex. The heavens are above, away from the earth, up, large, expansive, the centrifugal force, that power which draws away and dissipates—yin. The earth is solid, contracted, comparatively dense, holding by gravity those things created out of its substance and drawing toward it the finer forces found in outer space—yang. However, we realize that by scientific theory the earth, planets, and other "condensations" of celestial energy were created by the "heavens" and that the power to generate enormous amounts of matter from energy makes outer space, appearing to be so empty and expansive, a very yang entity. So we can speak of the heavens as being physically yin but metaphysically yang. We must, therefore, be aware of whether we are speaking of quantitative or qualitative factors when using yin and yang designations. In Chinese medicine, for instance, the solid organs such as the heart, kidneys, pancreas and liver are classified as yin. Although solid is a yang quality, the designation in Chinese medicine refers to the subtle qualities rather than to the quantitative aspect. Except for designating contraction as yin and expansion as yang, Chinese medicine agrees with macrobiotic assignations of these tendencies. If the components which make up the two Chinese characters for yin and yang are interpreted literally they mean "the shady side of a hill" for yin and "the sunny side of the hill" for yang.[3]

To return to the Genesis story, we find continued reference to various yin and yang qualities during the first moments of creation. In Genesis 1 : 3 the quality of light is created to balance the "darkness." We now have heavens and earth, affected by two other manifestations of yin and yang, darkness and light. Darkness is yin, light is yang. Most land animals are diurnal, active (yang) in the daytime, while they sleep (yin) at night. Our condition reflects our environment. When we get beyond this point in the Genesis story the analysis begins to break down because of the Old Testament understanding that the sky and earth are surrounded by water. When we look up on a clear day we can understand why. The sky is blue, like the sea. This water is "the deep" over which God's Spirit moved. The cosmology becomes somewhat confused in verse 6 when the firmament is created. The Hebrew word translated as "firmament" means platform. This "platform" as it is refined into heaven in verses 7 and 8 stands in opposition to earth, created in a separate act from the waters. The vegetation is created as the first of earth's living creatures, more yin than the mobile, active animals. This sequence of creation is similar to the "spiral of creation" in macrobiotic literature. The dominant celestial lights are created—the sun, bright, hot, creative energy, (yang), to rule the day, (yang), and the moon, passive and reflective, (yin), to rule the night, (yin). In fairness to this discussion it should be noted that the recognition by the Genesis writer of the essential qualities of the "heavens" and the "earth" constitute the incidence of that author's awareness of those qualities. Whether or not that awareness was present in other verses can only be deduced with the danger of projecting this writer's awareness on the writings of another. Such interpretation is tempting.

The most obvious reference to yin and yang qualities occurs in the Book of Ecclesiasticus, written around the year 180 B.C. and probably the oldest of the group of books in the Apocrypha, those writings from the period between the Old Testament and the New. This book was influenced by Greek thought to a great extent and, perhaps, the mention of created things being composed of pairs is also a specific borrowing from Greek thought. At any rate, the author specifically says, "All things go in pairs, one the opposite of the other. He has made nothing incomplete. One thing supplements the virtues of another," (Ecclesiasticus 42:24, 25). In a similar quote he says, "Look upon all the works of the most high. They, likewise, are in pairs, one the opposite of the other," (Ecclesiasticus 33:15). In this quote he is comparing the created order with the specific manifestations of good and evil, life and death, the sinner and the godly, mentioned in the previous verse.

It is the purpose of yin/yang theory not only to describe specific phenomena, but to equip the student of this theory to go and do likewise. Everything this side of the eternal One may be interpreted in terms of its relative yinness/yangness and which quality seems to dominate in relation to other phenomena. Thus, every passage of the Bible could be analyzed and interpreted. This activity can be fruitful as practice for seeing the manifestation of these qualities in everyday life and, through constant awareness of the ever-changing manifestation, to respond accordingly. The ability to respond (responsibility) is basic to macrobiotic philosophy and that ability is dependent upon having a fit body—physically, emotionally, and intellectually. The balance intrinsic to fitness may be attained by application of the universal principles and yin/yang theory. To do this requires a knowledge of those concepts which, although it can be learned intellectually to some extent, is a knowledge which must be lived with and experienced for some time before its application becomes second nature. However, this application is necessary for anyone who professes to be a practicing macrobiotic and is, in fact, what differentiates a macrobiotic from a non-macrobiotic person. Diet is such an obvious aspect of macrobiotic practice what it is often assumed that the food is what really demonstrates macrobiotic commitment. It is *understanding* the qualities of the food and the effect of consuming food possessing those qualities which really makes one macrobiotic. In theory a macrobiotic person could eat any food and still be a macrobiotic. However, understanding the effect of consuming just any food would prevent any responsible person from creating the imbalance produced by chaotic eating habits and the resulting diminished ability to judge the qualities of the food consumed.

We are assured by macrobiotic authors that attaining the necessary knowledge is not difficult, although we must take such statements on good faith as we try to figure out relative yinness and yangness in things not specifically mentioned by them.

> The yin-yang principle is simple. Fundamental to it is the assumption that the elements of nature are ephemeral and that, once aware of this, we must conduct our lives accordingly. These two forces are always opposite and antagonistic, and yet at the same time they are complementary, for they are forever combining and cooperating, both within the body and without. Thus the principle of Yin and Yang developed in the Orient is one of "dualistic monism."[4]

In speaking of the yin/yang principle Herman Aihara states:

> This is our guiding compass. It shows us our direction in life in much the same way a North-South compass shows us geographical direction. The yin-yang "unifying" principle is a useful tool for us. It can help us find our position in the infinite universe and it can also lead us to health and happi-

> ness by enabling us to analyze the foods we eat and their effects on our bodies and minds.[5]

I would refer the inquiring reader to any of the many full discussions in macrobiotic literature of the manifestation of yinness/yangness. Perusal of those simple charts and descriptions will soon suggest the gist of this concept so central to macrobiotic philosophy.[6]

The next step comes in observing these relative tendencies in daily life in objects with which we deal, situations in which we find ourselves, and people with whom we relate. It is particularly interesting to notice the ease with which difficulties may be resolved when, if other conditions permit, we adopt the opposite and complementary tendency as our approach. The aggressive (yang) person cannot fail to respond more favorably to a passive (yin) response than to an equally aggressive one. *Opposites* are complementary. The well worn adage of the business world, "The customer is always right!" is the result of someone's discovering the truth of the complementarity of opposites represented by the mutual attraction of yin and yang and the mutual repulsion of yang and yang, yin and yin. This lesson has also been learned easily by anyone who has ever played with Scotty Dog magnets. When they are moved head to head the similar poles repel and the dog not being held jumps back. When moved head to tail they opposite poles attract and the dogs become stuck together. We even use the expression, "going at it head to head" in describing an argument, or "toe to toe" in referring to a boxing match.

A most obvious and beautiful occurrence of attraction of yin and yang is found in the universal necessity of male and female qualities and quantities in creating offspring. The mutual attraction between male and female in all but species with asexual reproduction mirrors the initial act of creation in the arising of heaven and earth, yin and yang, femaleness and maleness, in order that any further act of creation be made possible. The creation of man and woman in Genesis 1:27 is the creation of yang and yin as predominant tendencies incarnate. In the third chapter the creation of man and woman is not a simultaneous event Adam is created first then Eve, from Adam's rib, as a refinement of the original work. Adam means "man" or "mankind" in Hebrew; The word "Eve" has at least nine possible derivations so, unfortunately, does not simply mean "woman." Eve may mean "to live," however, in recognition of the life-bearing quality of womanhood. Woman and man, the dyad constituting humanity, reflecting the creative dyad of yin and yang which constitutes all phenomena may be seen together as an inseparable pair whenever we travel in the company of others. I have often thought how well the power of yin to attract yang, as woman and man, is demonstrated by the occupants of automobiles with so many containing a man and a woman. In all shapes, weights and colors, some with rather yin men and yang women, others with yang men and yin women, all attracted to each other to form that archetypic pair. Most seem totally oblivious to the universal significance of their choice.

Even in the spiritual life of saints and sages this primal necessity is made manifest. Many male and female saints of the Church have given each other spiritual strength and vitality—St. Francis of Assisi and St. Clare, St. John of the Cross and St. Theresa, St. Francis de Sales and St. Jeanne de Chantal, St. Vincent de Paul and Louise de Marillac, St. Benedict and his sister St. Scholastica, St. John Vianney and St. Philomena, The Beloved Disciple and Jesus' mother, Zechariah and Elizabeth.

In macrobiotic philosophy even the basic creative energy of the universe is understood to flow from two distinct directions, above and below. Thus that life force which emanates from the bosom of the universe intermingles relative to our place on this planet creating maleness and femaleness depending in what relative proportion that intermingling takes place.

It is the contention of this book that the seven universal principles of the infinite universe constitute basic macrobiotics and all interpretation of those principles is only expository and illustrative of their truths. Such interpretation need not be considered universally essential since all interpretation reflects the cultural bias of the interpreter. Universals are transcultural truths not dependent upon a particular cultural milieu for their validity. Do we find a similar explanation of the dual nature of vivifying energy in other literature or is this interpretation peculiar to macrobiotics? This understanding exists elsewhere, and is particularly apparent in biblical literature as well as Greek mythology. It is definitely not peculiar to macrobiotic literature and deserves a place in any interpretation. In fact, practical application of the seven universal principles in food preparation and yin/yang theory would be impossible without realizing that even the basic life force descends (yang) and ascends (yin) in relation to the surface of the earth.

Science recognizes several kinds of radiation which descend upon us from outer space among which are ultra violet rays in sunlight, cosmic radiation, and the plasma thrown off by the sun in solar flares which interacts with our inosphere as the aurora borealis. Science describes the radiation produced by the earth itself which envelops the planet as the Van Allen Radiation Belt, magnetic radiation which emanates from the earth's two poles (even the earth energy has two sources) and helps humans and animals to navigate, gravitational pull which exists as mutual attraction with the enormous mass of the earth being far more attractive.

A graphic description of the power of earth energy in Greek mythology occurs in the story of the wrestling match between Hercules and Antaeus. Antaeus is the son of Terra, the earth. When he is in contact with his mother he gains strength. At first Hercules throws Antaeus down on the ground only to discover that his opponent springs up totally renewed and undefeated. Finally Hercules holds Antaeus in the air to strangle him. Antaeus is weakened by lack of contact with mother earth.

Our bodies are made of earth matter, built up by the ingestion of things of the earth, composed of combinations of elements found on this planet. We are, as Paul describes us, "of the earth, earthy," (1 Corinthians 15:47) fashioned from the "dust of the ground," (Genesis 2:7). When Adam and Eve are sent East of

Eden God says, among other things, "In the sweat of your face you shall eat bread until you return to the gound, for out of it you were taken; you are dust and to dust you shall return," (Genesis 3:19). The cells of our bodies are part of the planetary substance and we are cells in the body of the earth.

In the teaching of Jesus the two vivifying and sustaining forces appear as "bread," and "bread from heaven," also called "bread of God," "bread of life," and "word of God." Bread is ingestible earth energy, made from grain, grown out of the earth, a principle food of the people of biblical times. It was the food upon which they "leaned" for nourishment and is referred to as "the staff of bread" (Ezekiel 4:16; 5:16; 14:13; Psalm 105:16) giving rise to its designation as "the staff of life." As basic physical sustenance bread is a fitting subject of petition in the Lord's Prayer, "give us this day our daily bread," but Jesus points out to Satan that more than this physical condensation of life energy is required for life: "Man shall not live by bread alone but by every word that proceeds from the mouth of God," (Matthew 4:4). Both that which arises from earth and that which descends from heaven are required for life.

In the Gospel of John the early Church's identification of the Christ as inseparable from all of creation—". . . all things were made through him, and without him was not anything made that was made," (John 1:3)—is also reflected in Jesus' reference to himself as bread, both earthly and heavenly. After the feeding of the five thousand Jesus is reported as admonishing his followers not ot be overly concerned with perishable bread (physical sustenance) but the heavenly bread, (spiritual sustenance): "Do not labor for the food which perishes but for the food which endures to eternal life..." (John 6:27a). Then begins a description referring to the manna in the wilderness, which was a physical food mysteriously appearing each morning for the sustenance of the Israelites when they were in the wilderness headed toward the promised land. Manna is an interesting combination of the earthly and heavenly in that it is described as having appeared as a result of God's promise to "rain bread from heaven."

> Our fathers ate manna in the wilderness; as it is written, "He gave them bread from heaven to eat." Jesus then said to them, "Truly, truly, I say to you it was not Moses who gave you the bread from heaven. For the bread of God is that which comes down from heaven, and gives life to the world." They said to him, "Lord, give us this bread always."
>
> Jesus said to them, "I am the bread of life; he who comes to me shall not hunger; and he who believes in me shall never thirst." (John 6: 31–35)

> "I am the living bread which came down from heaven; if anyone eats of this bread, he will live forever; and the bread which I shall give for the life of the world is my flesh." (John 6: 51)

For the Christian believer, the earthly and heavenly creative forces are identified with the Christ. In particular the unifying of both aspects is effected and celebrated in the Eucharist, the ceremonial thanksgiving, in which the believer understands the Christ to be present in the elements of food and drink, bread and wine. The Mass, Holy Communion, Lord's Supper, Eucharist, whatever it is called in the various denominations within Christendom, is the celebration *par excellence* of the coming together of the earthly and the heavenly and is the principle act of worship in all denominations which observe the catholic (universal) tradition. "Earth's force" and "heaven's force" are central to Christian theology, too, although they are called by other names.

Biblical cosmology, in positing a three tiered universe with heaven above earth, establishes a model which easily accomodates to the use of descending and ascending "forces" in macrobiotic cosmology. The macrobiotic description does no violence to biblical belief. Since there is ample confirmatory evidence from science, mythology, and the Bible for the existence of both down ward and upward "forces" this particular discussion should serve as an example to any interpreter of macrobiotics not to relegate a particular interpretation to only one school of thought. The interpretations of the seven principles found in mainstream macrobiotic literature are, in many cases, ancient understandings; philosophical concepts, as well as practical way of life suggestions, must be tried on for validity.

George Ohsawa's principle of "non credo," recently has been reflected on bumper stickers proclaiming, "Question Authority," (by whose authority the author of the bumper sticker makes his proclamation we are not told). This principle must be applied by each of us as an "owned" macrobiotic philosophy is refined in the crucible of experience. Work in faith development by James Fowler and John Westerhoff has borne out the necessity for such "trying on" of new concepts and behavior in the important selection process which results in the construction our own (owned) understandings. Their interesting work in tracing the evolution of mature faith places the questioning of authority dead center in the process. Their suggestion, therefore, is that institutions dealing with such processes foster an atmosphere of open questioning so that the growth to maturity will not be impeded. Macrobiotics has shown great wisdom in this regard; the church's image is not so fortunate.

The central symbol of Christendom, the cross, is recognized in Sunday school classes and classical theology as representing the coming together of the vertical (yin) and the horizontal (yang), ascending (yin) and descending (yang), left and right. As the symbol for the atonement the cross also represents the resolution of opposing forces in a still-point at its center. It has special significance for the Christian since it was on a cross that the master died, but, as a symbol for reality, it joins those other symbols of world religions in representing the harmonizing of opposites.[7]

The well-known authority on world religions, Huston Smith, states the following about the cross:

> Two kinds of resolution are represented. The first of these is *the union of complements*. Things that are complementary differ from each other, and the differences can produce tensions and even open warfare. But the differences can also

"come together," as the convergence of the horizontal and vertical arms indicate. In intersecting, the arms of the vertical cross form, as it were, a Western yin-yang.[8]

The horizontal arms of the cross represents the earthly, our relationships, community, humanitarian activities, all that is seen by us as being between us and the horizons of our life space. The vertical beam bisects the moment, represents the inbreaking of the eternal found only in the moment, supports the horizontal from both below and above. The cross symbolizes the moment in which we find ourselves, the eternal now. Each of us has a unique moment since no two things are identical, and how each lives that moment depends upon how each decides to carry that cross. There are no two personal crosses the same, no two constellations of left and right, above and below, yin and yang. Jesus' call to take up our cross and follow him is a call to personal responsibility for our own reality.

Once a man entered a cross-maker's shop to exchange his cross for one which fit better. He unshouldered his cross by the door and asked if he could try on some of the models on display around the shop. The cross maker advised him to take his time and to make his choice carefully since he would be carrying his new cross for the rest of his life. He was also advised that there was no market for used crosses and that he would not be allowed an allowance on the old one as a trade-in. The first cross he tried was too short and required him to bend backward too much in order for it to reach the ground. The second had arms which were so long that they tended to catch on things both on the ground and overhead. Another just fit his shoulder all wrong, its vertical was too wide and cut into his shoulder blade. He worked his way around the store, but each cross had some uncomfortable aspect. His desperation grew as he reached the last cross. When he tried it on he knew that this one was the cross he had been looking for. It was just right. He asked the price. "It's free!" the cross-maker said. "How can that be?" the man replied. "I know that the cross business is your livelihood. You can't possibly give them away." Then he learned what he had done: "That one is free, because it is the one you carried in and left by the door."

Where is God in all this? Does yin/yang theory explain away the numinous and depersonalize the *mysterium tremendum*? A key to answering these questions is found in the Gospel According to Thomas, a gospel found at Nag Hamadi in Egypt in 1945 interpreting Jesus mission and ministry in the language and imagery of Gnostic Christianity, influenced by Greek culture, and dating originally from around A.D. 140. This early Christian book reports Jesus as saying, "If they ask you: What is the sign of your Father in you?' say to them, 'It is a movement and a rest,'" (90: 4–6).[9] Here we find an interpretation of the presence of the One in history, in the now, as the two complementary opposites which comprise all that is. Yin/yang theory identifies, localizes and makes specific the most basic sphere of activity of "your Father within you." Heaven and Earth, polarity, movement and rest are the primal tendencies of the world of phenomena where the first promptings of the Spirit are displayed.

If we look at a dominant theme in the New Testament descriptive of the presence of the One we find numerous references to love. "God is love," proclaims the writer of the First Epistle of John (4: 16b). "Love is the fulfilling of the law," states Paul in Romans 13: 10. Jesus told his hearers that all of the law and the prophets (the whole writings of the Old testament) can be hung on the two commandments, "Love the Lord your God with all your heart, with all your soul, with all your mind. . . . Love your neighbor as yourself," (Matthew 22: 37–39). Love is central to the message of the New Testament and to the mission and achievement of Jesus. His life is the ultimate demonstration of the life of love. In the crucifixion is the living out of the statement, "There is no greater love than this, that a man should lay down his life for his friends," (John 15: 13). John even describes love as the mode of being which enables the unitive experience, conscious union with the One: "God himself dwells in us if we love one another," (1 John 4: 12).

Given the danger of using this word in a world inundated with identification of love with "falling in love," there is still much to be learned in examining this unifying activity and state of consciousness. Since God is love, love is a universal. It is as universal as the arising of polar opposites. There could be no cosmos without it. Love is found within the basic creative tendencies of yin and yang and is, therefore, the power of attraction by which one tendency is drawn to interaction with the other. Love is, as George Ohsawa has said, "so vast as to make opposites complementary." To carry the description of love to the level of atomc activity may seem demeaning and a depersonalization of this highly personal emotion, but what manifests as emotion on the human level can be described as manifesting as simple attraction on the nuclear level.

Next to Dali's magnificent painting of The Crucifixion of St. John of the Cross in the Kelvingrove Gallery in Glasgow, there hangs a small study and description by Dali of what he calls "nuclear mysticism." In a dream he saw an atom split apart and tetrahedrons of energy fly from it.[10] In Salvadore Dali's dream he came to understand that Christ is the "power which binds the universe together." It was in discussing this dream with a person acquainted with St. John of the Cross' sketch of a vision of the crucifixion (from which St. John gets his name) that Dali was introduced to that sketch. It became a study for his painting.

This binding force, the Word of God first spoken, "with God at the beginning, and through him all things came to be; no single thing was created without him," (John 1:2) is identified by Dali and the writer of John as none other than the power incarnate in Jesus of Nazareth: the creative and vivifying power of love.

Within the human condition this state of being is demonstrated as "the will to extend one's self for the purpose of nurturing one's own or another's spiritual growth,"[11] or in the words of Brother David Steindl-Rast, "Love is a wholehearted 'yes' to belonging."[12] Love contains the quality of affirming, willing, doing—a yang quality. But as expected since every front has a back, love also enters (yin) in a spontaneous infilling of Grace, unearned, involuntary and surprising. Suddenly, awareness of unity in the midst of diversity is just there. The yin quality of love is the receiving side of giving/receiving; it is openness to listening.

Both sides of love are graphically portrayed in the Gospel accounts of Jesus' life. Even at the moment of conception there is the descent (yang) of the Holy Spirit into the young virgin Mary whose response to Gabriel's announcement is an appropriately yin, "as you have spoken, so be it," (Luke 1:38). Jesus responds to the descent of the dove (yang) at his baptism by a retreat (yin) into solitude and silence (yin) to the emptiness (yin) of the wilderness. In Toynbee's designations the "challenge" of the Baptism is balanced by the "response" of the desert experience. The public ministry is characterized by the yang activity, noise, and "press of the crowd" (Luke 8:19) balanced by sometimes successful attempts at solitude, retreat, and prayer. An example of the latter is found in Matthew 14 when the extremely busy and eventful (yang) feeding of the five thousand is immediately followed by going "up the hillside to pray alone," (verse 23). The horizontal (yang) activity demonstrating love of neighbor is followed by the vertical (yin) receptivity in solitude of the love of God in prayer. Little children are received into Jesus' arms and pointed to as characteristic of those in the Kingdom (Mark 10:15, 16) and those same arms drive into the street the money changers and those who sold sacrificial animals in the Temple, (Matthew 21:10–17; Mark 11:11–14; Luke 19:45–46). The mouth which announces eternal life in the coming of the Kingdom (Mark 1:15), curses the fig tree to death. (Matthew 21:19). Both sides of love incarnate are portrayed throughout the short ministry of Jesus and culminate in the willingness (yin) to be crucified and the invincibility (yang) of life over death, light over darkness, demonstrated in the resurrection. The story of the early Church's life begins in earnest with the descent (yang) of the Holy Spirit at Pentecost upon the waiting and receptive (yin) disciples.

The Biblical acounts equate ebb and flow, receiving and giving, acceptance and anger, movement and rest with the operation of the One Spirit at work in creation. There is an implicit understanding of the need for balance as one quality moves toward its opposite in that inexorable cosmic dance described by the seven principles. The Infinite One is there in the two as the two complete the trinitarian nature of all things by creating the manifestation of their interaction. Father, Son, and Holy Spirit; father, mother, child; light and dark, one day; challenge, response, event; the two become lost in the three. In endless swirling and interplay we join what Ram Dass has called "the only dance there is." It is the dance of the universe and of the One in whose sea of life we live. In that moment where the peace which passes understanding is found, at the junction of left and right, up and down, we remember who it is we are, "but a mist, here for awhile and then dispersing." We remember that it *is* more blessed to give than to receive because in giving we lose the memory of the appearance of the mask called personality and regain the memory of our original face created before God "laid the foundation of the earth," (Job 38: 4).

The prayer attributed to Saint Francis of Assisi, one of the most popular in Christendom, calls us to active participation in the dance of complementary opposites and sums up this chapter well:

> Lord, make us instruments of your peace. Where there is hatred, let us sow love; where there is injury, pardon; where there is discord, union; where there is doubt, faith; where there is despair, hope; where there is darkness, light; where there is sadness, joy; grant that we may not so much seek to be consoled as to console; to be understood as to understand; to be loved as to love. For it is in giving that we receive; it is in pardoning that we are pardoned; and it is in dying that we are born to eternal life.

---

[1] Davies, *God and the New Physics,* p. 228.
[2] Toynbee, *A Study of History,* p. 89.

[3] See *The Yellow Emperor's Classic of Internal Medicine,* Ilza Veith, translator, pp. 13–18, for a full discussion. George Ohsawa's understanding of yin as expansive and yang as contractive has caused no small amount of consternation among some yin/yang theorists who believe that in so doing he did such violence to traditional Chinese medicine that he cut macrobiotics free from its rightful place as an inheritor of that tradition.

[4] Muramoto, *Healing Ourselves,* p. 8.

[5] Aihara, *Seven Basic Macrobiotic Principles,* p. 5.

[6] See Kushi, *The Book of Macrobiotics,* pp. 7–9; Muramoto, *Healing Ourselves,* pp. 8–9; Aihara, *Seven Basic Macrobiotic Principles,* pp. 5–7; Ohsawa, *The Book of Judgment,* Chapter 2; Esko and Esko, *Macrobiotic Cooking for Everyone,* Chapter 1.

[7] For a description of seven symbols used by world religions see p. 15, *The Book of Macrobiotics,* Kushi.

[8] Smith, *Forgotten Truth,* p. 26.

[9] *The Gospel According to Thomas,* p. 29.

[10] These pyramids with triangular bases are familiar to anyone acquainted with the writings of Buckminster Fuller. He demonstrated that a sphere is made up of them with their apices at the center. This fact may be seen most obviously in Fuller's Geodesic Dome composed of the bases of those tetrahedrons.

[11] Peck, *The Road Less Traveled,* p. 81.

[12] Steindl-Rast, *Gratefulness, The Heart of Prayer,* p. 206.

Chapter 8

Bible Food

"O taste and see that the Lord is good!"
(Psalm 34 : 8)

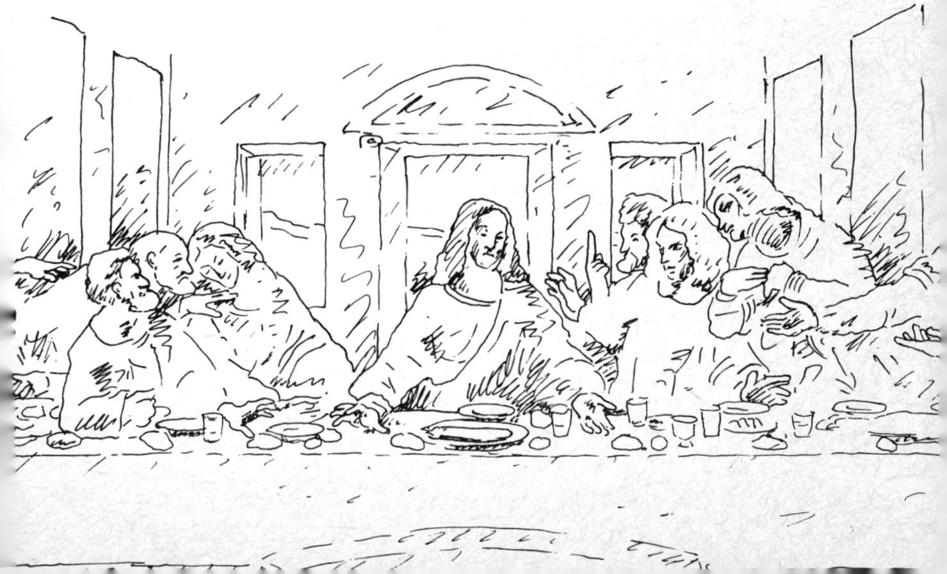

THE TITLE FOR THIS CHAPTER WAS PROVIDED by a friend with whom I was discussing macrobiotics. He is well acquainted with the writings of the Bible, and we were discussing the diet of biblical people. I listed the standard dietary guidelines of macrobiotics for our latitude: 25% vegetables, 10–15% beans and sea vegetables, 5% soup, 5–10% fish, shellfish, fruits, nuts, and other foods, 50–60% whole grains. We talked about the centrality of grain in these guidelines and suddenly he said, "That's Bible food!"

The standard dietary guidelines of macrobiotics do, in fact, describe the food of the people of the Bible. These guidelines also outline the diet of all peoples who have not lost touch with the traditional food of their culture. Except for the extreme conditions of the polar and equatorial regions, humanity has sustained itself on the simple, whole foods, described in these guidelines. In the extreme climates the dietary proportions have been altered by any number of appropriate factors rendering the virtually all-meat diet of the Greenland Eskimo and the abundantly fruitarian cuisine of the equatorial islanders the natural and "macrobiotic" diet for them.

Macrobiotics is far more than diet, however. The Seven Universal Principles of the Infinite Universe form a philosophical basis for a way of life and a way of understanding. They put all things in perspective, not only food. The Unique Principle, or the Order of the Universe, is the macrobiotic's "guiding compass," as Herman Aihara points out.[1] This encompassing understanding is used by the macrobiotic for guidance in areas other than diet. However, the compass points to certain foods as appropriate to certain seasons and geographical locations, and, three times a day, the application of the Laws of Change of the Infinite Universe[2] appear at mealtime. As a result those not fully acquainted with macrobiotic philosophy assume that macrobiotics is little more than a diet. This misunderstanding gives rise to the inevitable series, "Can you eat this? Can you eat that?" The fact is you can eat anything which fits in the oral orifice, but would you want to? Recently I read about a man who ate his Jeep!

Modern macrobiotics, though, *did* begin with an understanding of the application of yin/yang theory to diet by a Doctor, Sagen Ishizuka, who discovered the importance of the sodium/potassium ratio in creating balance. His work of 100 years ago demonstrated to him the balancing power of brown rice, and he came to understand that food is the best medicine. His student, George Ohsawa, named this science of foods for health and happiness "macrobiotics." He recognized the antagonistic complementarity of potassium and sodium, potassium producing an expansive effect, sodium producing a contractive, and thus began the elaboration of the application of yin/yang theory to diet and the beginning of modern macrobiotics. The work of Ohsawa and many of his early students has, naturally enough, left macrobiotic philosophy and dietary recommendations with a distinct oriental interpretation. As stated earlier, the basic principles are universal in application. They are only now being interpreted out of other cultural traditions as the universalization of macrobiotics takes place.

The roots of macrobiotics are deep in the cultural soil of Japan. A brief look at the history of the movement may help our appreciation of how both East and West created the dynamic which spawned the genesis of Dr. Ishizuka's work, and how it was the West to which George Ohsawa was drawn as if by a magnet.

During the period from 1540 to 1640 there was a Western presence in Japan and that presence was not without influence. However, in 1640 Japan was closed to Western presence until 1853 and Commodore Matthew Perry's arrival in Tokyo harbor. By the time of Perry's arrival the West was industrialized while Japan was still agrarian. Perry declared that the country would be open and who was there to argue with his cannon and muskets? After the signing of an appropriate treaty there began the importation of Western industrial and agricultural techniques as well as the Western understanding of medicine. Sagen Ishizuka was born at this time.

Prime in the arsenal of Western medicine was Pasteur's notion of the bacterial genesis of disease and the attending primary focus on destroying these organisms. The science of nutrition was also evolving with work being done in Germany on analyzing various foods for constituent nutrients and the necessity of these nutrients in the human diet. These early results showed that protein was of great importance; thus began an emphasis on protein-dense foods such as meat and eggs. Quality was not a consideration; all food was organically grown at that time, and the constituent nutrients were the prime concern, not the nature of the source of those nutrients, (an error still very much in evidence today). Studies also showed that carbohydrates were an energy source; thus simple, quick carbohydrates like sugar must be most desirable. Today we know the role sugar plays in dental caries, behavioral problems in the young, in leaching calcium from the system, in causing pancreatic insufficiency. We know that the prison population consumes five times the 130 pounds per year of the average American, and still one sees advertisements touting sugar as an appropriate energy source. 19th Century Japan found these early days of allopathy so convincing that it declared the Western approach to be the official medicine of the country in 1873. A medical school was established at Tokyo to teach this approach and it was this school from which Sagen Ishizuka graduated.

At the age of thirty Ishizuka became ill and could find no relief within the Western approach, so began studying traditional medidine, especially the volume known as *The Yellow Emperor's Classic of Internal Medicine*. One particular statement in the book fascinated Dr. Ishizuka, "The primary cause of disease is improper diet." The first approach recommended in the volume was a ten day rice gruel fast; if that failed to bring results then medicinal herbs *and* food were used. In the event that the second approach failed acupuncture and moxabustion treatments were recommended. The first approach and the heart of the second approach was dietary. Dr. Ishizuka began several years of experimentation on recuperating soldiers, formulated a theory to guide his experiments, and in 1898, published an enormous tome entitled, *A Chemical/Nutritional Theory of Long Life,* the first macrobiotic book. His summary of the ponderous volume published the following year received wider attention and detailed his theory: (1) The most important factor in human health is the proper relation between Sodium and Potassium salts. (2) The primary determinant of this proportion is the food we eat and liquid we consume. (3) Food is the primary cause of disease. (4) Dietary therapy is the appropriate therapy.

In specific application his theory is "cerealism:" that cereal grains are the staple food of human beings. A look at cultures worldwide confirms the truth of this assertion, whether the rice of the orient, the buckwheat of the Russians and Eastern Europeans, the millet of the Africans, the oats and barley of Northern Europeans, the maize of the Mayans and Aztecs, or the ubiquitous wheat, rye, spelt, and other grass seeds. Grain is found sustaining human life in all but the most extreme climatic and geographical conditions.

Another aspect of Dr. Ishizuka's theory still very much in evidence in macrobiotic recommendations is the idea of "shin-do-fu-ji," meaning "the body and the earth are not two," or "the human being and his natural environment are one." Physically, we are transormations of the natural environment; thus, to be happy and healthy we should consume the foods which grow in our immediate environment. Dr. Ishizuka saw that not only are we one with our environment, but each person is an integrated whole; everything we say or do is interrelated. A change in any part of our reality affects all other parts. His teaching was wholistic.

In the early part of the 20th Century Dr. Ishizuka had gathered students around him, before his death in 1910. His legacy has been expanded upon and internationally recognized through the work of George Ohsawa who took Ishizuka's teachings as the basis for his own work. Ohsawa's mission took him to the West and eventually to the United States. His students have carried on and built upon his teaching and refined its application to those of Western physical heritage. However, all of the present teachers have kept the heart of macrobiotics as described by Ohsawa: (1) The natural state of the human being is health. (2) This health or lack of it is no accident; we are responsible for our health according to the laws of cause and effect. (3) One of the important factors in determining health is the food we eat. (4) In choosing our food we should be aware of our environment (shin-do-fu-ji) which means, for the most part, a diet based upon grains, beans, and vegetables. (5) Every aspect of our functioning is related to every other. (6) The entire cosmos is an integrated system. The above principles are either explicitly stated, implied, or such a fact of life as to make their ėlaboration unnecessary in biblical writing. With reference to the first principle: both the Old and New Testaments view disease as unnatural. In the former it is seen as punishment or the result of behavior not in accord with divine will. In Jesus' ministry it is seen as occasion for the manifestation of divine power, not due to the sins of one's ancestors, but the result of negative influences sometimes personalized as evil spirits, sometimes seen as the result of not practicing those characteristics of life in the kingdom described in the Sermon on the Mount. Occurrence of the second principle is apparent as Job's friends attempt to point out to him that he is responsible for his state of affairs. Jesus asks many whom he heals, "Do you want to be healed?" After the healing he then tells them, "Your faith has made you whole," and advises them to "Go, sin no more." Responsibility for both the onset of disease, the healing, and the future condition rests with the individual. Principles 3 and 4 are implied. Except for the wealthy the daily diet was locally produced food, grain-based, with the consumption of fruits and vegetables in season or preserved by salting or drying. Of course, all food was organically grown in a chemical-free environment. Principles 5 and 6 are explicit in the biblical writers' understanding of the unity of creation as discussed in detail in Chapter 1. This belief centers around the procession of all things from one creative power (an Old Testament understanding) and the incarnation of that essential vitality in human form demon strating the eternal unity between creator and creation (the New Testament message).

Point number 4, above, is that which most characterizes the acquisition, preparation, and consumption of food in native cultures. It would not be necessary to admonish what we consider a primitive people to be aware of their environment and the food they choose. Lack of awareness could mean disease, famine, or possible extinction. All people living a natural life style are aware that their bodies and the earth are not two. It is "progress' and "civilization" which tears us from our roots and require us to work at remembering that "You shall gain your bread by the sweat of your brow until you return to the ground; for from it you were taken. Dust you are, to dust you shall return," (Genesis 3: 19). People of the polar regions follow migrating herds, native Americans of the Northwest know the time when salmon are returning from the sea, and prehistoric peoples of the flood planes of the Nile planted their grains, moved on, then returned at harvest. All whose lives depend upon the natural elements see their lives as inextricably bound up with the natural order.

Today there are urban people who descend by elevator from their apartments to the parking garage below ground, ride in air conditioned cars to the parking garage of the office building where they work and ascend by elevator to the controlled atmosphere of their workplace. Is it any wonder that they develop agoraphobia (the fear of being in an open space), bizarre degenerative diseases unimaginable a generation ago, and must be admonished to be aware of the foods they select? In fact, the enormous popularity of books on diet and cooking may not so much be an expression of America's desire to improve our diet as an admission of just how far away we have drifted from a natural understanding of such things. We need guidelines to lead us to what we really should have known all along.

Macrobiotics offers such dietary suggestions and rightfully claims that these flexible guidelines which take into consideration geographical setting, lattitude, climate and lifestyle represent the traditional diet of all peoples everywhere. The way to prove such a claim is to look at the dietary patterns of a traditional culture and compare them with the macrobiotic suggestions. Archaeological work done on the floodplanes of the Nile by a team representing Southern Methodist University, the Geological

Survey of Egypt, and the Polish Academy of Sciences has unearthed evidence that crops of wheat, barley, lentils, chick-peas, capers and dates were being raised there 18,500 years ago. This sets the date for the beginning of agriculture back some 8,000 years before most textbooks say it began. In southern Africa grinding stones have been found which were in use 36,000 years ago, but there is no way to be sure that they were used for an agricultural product rather than a foraged food. The researchers *are* sure that the grains wheat and barley, and the legumes lentils and chick-peas were grown by the people of Wadi Kubbaniya. In a fascinating report on the dig in the November, *Science 82* periodical, the American and Polish archaeologists report,

> These Nile sites indicate not that Wadi Kubbaniya was an isolated occurrence but rather that the use of cereals was widespread, occuring among diverse cultural groups and persisting as an important economic activity for at least 6,000 years after the time of Wadi Kubbaniya.[3]

Included in this report are maps showing the presence of cultivated millet and soybeans in eastern Asia 5,750 years ago; wheat, barley, peas, and legumes at the eastern end of the Mediterranean 9,000 years ago, and corn and beans in Central American 9,000 years ago. A remarkable aspect of this study is that it demonstrates how slowly staple foods change. The wheat, barley peas and legumes found to exist 9,000 years ago at the eastern end of the Mediterranean were still the staple food of the people of the Bible some 5,000 to 7,000 years later, and, wherever they can be grown, grains and beans to this day comprise the principle food of traditional lifestyles. This basic dietary pattern is even described by Aztecs in a conversation with Franciscan missionaries recorded in 1524 under the title, "What we know about our Gods."

> It was their doctrine that they [the gods] provide our subsistence, all that we eat and drink, that which maintains life: corn, beans, amaranth, sage.[4]

All the more remarkable is the comparison of this stability with the radical changes in dietary patterns experienced in the United States. In the sixty years betwen 1910 and 1970 annual per capita consumption of flour and cereal products has dropped from three hundred pounds per person to less than one hundred fifty, while total meat consumption has risen from one hundred thirty six pounds to one hundred sixty eight. Citrus consumption, only a rare treat in 1910, rose to over ninety pounds. Soft drinks, another specialty item in the late 19th century, are consumed today as the principle beverage in the United States with each person consuming, on the average, forty one gallons per year. Frozen dairy products, eaten at an average rate of two pounds per year in 1910, now are consumed at a rate of over thirty pounds.

There are several reasons why these figures are important. They represent a retreat from the food which has traditionally sustained our ancestors, which comprised the building blocks of their physical nature and created the blood quality which produced their psychological/emotional nature. There has been an increase of many thousandfold in the consumption of food which has been chemicalized, fractured, precooked, frozen, devitalized, and refined. Is it possible to consume fractured, devitalized food and not take on these qualities ourselves? To what degree are we what we eat? There is no definitive answer to that question, because there is no way to objectively measure all aspects, quantitative and qualitative, of a food and its effects. Western science, guided by its own methodology, gives no credence to qualitative factors but only those which can be measured and quantified such as nutrient content, caloric value, liquid content, weight, etc. Surely all can agree that what we eat becomes us except for that which is excreted by the organs of elimination.

The phrase, "You are what you eat," is the title of a book by Victor H. Lindlahr first published in 1940 and reprinted many times. Mr. Lindlahr had a television program by the same name and used the phrase as his sign-off at the end of each show. Having seen the show as a child, the phrase has stayed with me and now has taken on literal value as I have come to understand the wisdom it contains in the light of macrobiotics. It is common parlance to refer to someone as "beefy," "chicken," "a turkey," "a pig," or to liken them to some other animal because they exhibit a physical resemblance or behavior associated with that animal. The announcer in the radio advertisement for full cut blue jeans makes the claim that ". . . nature changes our shape as we grow older, and it's not because of too many Broncoburgers, either!" The jeans are designed to have "a 'skosh' more room in the seat and thigh." The reason this extra room is needed is because the American diet produces a body which, frankly, is "beefy." When this commercial is followed by one for a fast-food hamburger chain it is difficult not to make associations. As we observe the somatotypes of peoples whose dietary patterns do not include large amounts of animal food we do not find the need for "a 'skosh' more room in the seat and thigh." Such traditional diets are also associated with people who are physically more active than the average American, but the commercial for these jeans is always set in a physically active enrironment with the announcer posing as a tennis coach, gymnastics instructor, or health club operator. When a human baby is nourished on food for baby cows and then grows up eating that same food—curded, frozen, homogenized, and pasteurized—on the average, one hundred pounds each year, is it really far-fetched to assume that qualities peculiar to that animal will *not* manifest in that person? Do we really think that the only thing received from that food is quantitative nutrient value? Without delving into why a leading chicken grower who appears in his own television commercials looks so much like a chicken, or whether egg eating produces a desire to be "in a shell," or if peanutbutter eaters tend to feel "stuck" in life, raising this subject is intended to give the reader an opportunity to do some enjoyable observing. Think of the qualities of the animals whose diets predominate in certain foods and see if those qualities do not appear in people whose diets are also heavily composed of those foods. Also observe whether or not the people take on the qualities of the foodstuffs, themselves, animal *or* vegetable when considerable quantities of those foods are consumed regularly. You may agree that "we are what we eat."

Most religions know at least that what we eat has an effect on who we are. Thus, there are dietary guidelines in most of the world's religions, sometimes highly evolved and complex, sometimes limited only to suggestions that fasting—a dietary approach to cleansing and spirituality—be practiced at stipulated times of the year. Food for spiritual development is recognized in the Eastern religions, and in Buddhism there are strictures against meat, sweets and spices with such prohibitions stated on signs in monastery courtyards. In India, Sankhya and Vedantic philosophy recognize three qualities of manifestation—*rajas* (activity), *tamas* (inertia), and *sattva* (harmonious balance). Spiritual masters advise their followers against eating food of tamastic or rajasic quality and to consume only sattvic food. Similar prohibitions also exist in Islam as the British found out when both Islamic and Hindu soldiers refused to bite the ends off their pork fat lubricated cartridges thus beginning the Sepoy Mutiny of 1857–58 and the eventual loss of the East India Company's right to rule India.

The native Meso-American cultures may have come closer to saying, "you are what you eat," in their numerous references to maize as the mother of humankind. *The Song of Chicomecoatl, Our Mother Goddess* addresses her as Seven Cobs of Corn:

> Oh Seven Cobs of Corn . . . arise now, awaken . . . You are Our Mother! You would leave us orphans; go now to your house, Tlalocan. Oh Seven Cobs of Corn . . . arise now, awaken . . . You are Our Mother! You would leave us orphans; go now to your house, Tlalocan.[5]

The native North Americans also celebrated their sustenance ritualistically. In a Seneca Thanksgiving Address, corn, beans, and squash—the three cultivated foods of the Iroquois—are referred to in a statement typical of the recognition that the body and the earth are not two.

> When they emerge from the earth we see them. They bring us contentment. They come again with the change of the wind. And they strengthen our breath. . . . Those who take care of them every day asked, too, that they be sisters. And at that time there arose a relationship between them: we shall say "The Sisters, our sustenance," when we want to refer to them.[6]

The religious dietary restrictions with which the people of the West are most familiar are those of Judaism and Christianity. The logo identifying merchandise as Kosher is familiar to all food store shoppers. Fish is still a Friday feature in many school cafeterias and restaurants although the Roman Catholic Church no longer requires that abstention from meat be a Friday discipline. These strictures come from the Bible and Church tradition and are further examples of concern for diet on the part of world religions.

The dietary laws of Judaism find their source in the writings of the Old Testament where specific instructions can be quite complex, as a perusal of Leviticus 11, and Deuteronomy 14 will reveal. It was understood that humankind was permitted to eat plants: "God also said, 'I give you all plants bearing seed everywhere on earth, and every tree bearing fruit which yields seed: they shall be yours for food'," (Genesis 1:29). This statement was not modified in the laws of Moses. Permission to eat meat is recorded as coming immediately after the flood, the only restriction being that meat with blood in it was not to be eaten, (Genesis 9:3, 4). This information did not turn Noah into a total meat eater, however. He is described in 9:20 as "a man of the soil," and we are told that he set about planting a vineyard. The ninth chapter goes on to report the results of the abuse of the fermented product of that fruit. Some vegetarian writers take delight in pointing out that after meat eating is permitted the lifespan of Noah's descendants declined rapidly. Noah lived to 950 years, his son Shem lived only to 602. It should be mentioned also that Noah had Shem when he was 500, so Shem lived 100 years before the flood, thus had a solid vegetarian background. Shem's son, though, really suffered the degeneration induced by indulging in animal food and only lived to 438 years of age. His great, great grandson lived to only 239 and *his* great grandson lived to only 148. It was all downhill after "Broncoburgers."

Since the word "macrobiotic" in classical usage means "long lived," the fantastic figures quoted above are of particular interest. Just how long *did* people in biblical times expect to live? In the midst of that enigmatic passage about the "sons of the gods" and "the daughters of men" in Genesis 6: 1–4, the writer seems pretty certain in stating, "But the Lord said, 'My life-giving spirit shall not remain in man forever; he for his part is mortal flesh: he shall live for one hundred and twenty years." Allowing for the fact that one hundred twenty is a round number occuring also in Numbers 7: 86; 1 Kings 9: 14; 10: 10, it still must have represented a reasonable expectation for both the writer and the reader of that time. The writer of Ecclesiasticus tends to agree stating, "His span of life is at the most one hundred years," (18: 9). However, Psalm 90: 10a reckons life expectancy more within the limits accepted today, "The years of our life are threescore and ten, or even by reason of strenth fourscore." The ages of the kings of Israel and Judah are recorded faithfully and reflect ages nearer to the psalmist's estimate. But there are those tremendous figures ascribed to the quasi-immortal, legendary figures of Genesis quoted above as well as those of the Hebrew patriarchs also recorded in Genesis: Abraham, 175 (25: 7); Isaac, 180 (35: 28); Jacob, 147 (47: 28); Joseph, 110 (50: 22). We are told in Deuteronomy 34: 7, "Moses was one hundred twenty years old when he died; his sight was not dimmed nor had his vigor failed." At the time of the writing of Leviticus there were enough sixty plus year olds around to warrant placing a lower value on them presumably on the grounds of diminished usefulness. Chapter 27, verse 3–7 advises that a male between twenty and sixty is worth fifty shekels, but that he depreciates to only fifteen shekels when over sixty. Females also depreciate by two thirds from thirty shekels to ten. The biblical record holder is Methusaleh at 969 years (Genesis 5:27). In the classical use of the word he certainly was macrobiotic!

There is a mention of longevity in the secular literature of the New Testament period with an interesting interpretation. Flavius Josephus, a Pharisee by practice who had lived three years in an Essene community, was the great Jewish historian of his day. He has left us a detailed description of Essene practices, many of which seem reflected in the behavior of the disciples of Jesus' teaching, and in the customs of the early church. In his volume *The Wars of the Jews or The History of The Destruction of Jerusalem*, Book II, Chapter 8, Paragraph 10 he says of the Essenes,

> They are long-lived also, insomuch that many of them live above one hundred years, by means of the simplicity of their diet; nay, as I think, by means of the regular course of life they observe also.[7]

In Paragraph 5, we are told not only what they ate but how they took their meals: first they bathe in cold water, put on white robes used only for dining, spend some time in solitude (presumably to pray or meditate) and then,

> . . . go, after a pure manner, into the dining room as into a certain holy temple, and quietly set themselves down; upon which the baker lays them loaves in order; the cook also brings in a single plate of one sort of food, and sets it before every one of them; but a priest says grace before the meal and it is unlawful for anyone to taste of the food before grace be said.[8]

This description of peace and quiet, reverence and simplicity, is reflected in Michio Kushi's fifteen Principles of Cooking, especially the last principle,

> The atmosphere of the cooking and eating place should be

kept clean and quiet, and those who cook, serve, and eat should maintain a peaceful mind.[9]

Archaeological and historical evidence bears out the claim that biblical people were macrobiotic in the dietary sense as well as in being "long-lived." Their primary food was of vegetable origin with meat eaten only on special occasions such as religious feasts and family celebrations—all within present day macrobiotic guidelines for people living active lives in that climate and latitude. Genesis 1:29 gave permission to eat vegetable foods, and that passage was all that was required as a dietary guide to vegetarian fare. Animal quality food required very specific regulation, however, and the animal kingdom is divided up into four categories: animals (Leviticus 11:2), water creatures (Leviticus 11:9), birds (Leviticus 11:13), and winged insects (Leviticus 11:20). Although beasts which do not both divide the hoof and chew the cud are declared unclean by this rule of thumb, there *are* specific lists of unclean animals such as the one in Deuteronomy 14:6–8: the camel, the rock badger, the hare, and the swine. Animals which may be eaten are: ox, sheep, goat, hart, gazelle, roebuck, wild goat, ibex, antelope, and mountain sheep, (Deuteronomy 14:4). Among water creatures only those with both fins and scales may be eaten, (Deuteronomy 14:9, 10). Birds which are flesh eaters and scavengers are listed as unclean in both Leviticus and Deuteronomy. The Deuteronomy code makes all insects unfit for food, but the Leviticus list permits eating jumping insects such as crickets, locusts and grasshoppers. John The Baptizer, reported as making locusts and wild honey his food, must have been following the Leviticus list.

These laws were inherited by the early Christians whose first adherants, like the apostles, were practicing Jews. In fact, the resolution of problems posed by the dietary code to an increasingly gentile church is reported in the symbolic dream of Peter (Acts 10:9–16) in which a sheet containing all kinds of animals is lowered from heaven accompanied by a divine voice declaring them all fit for food. This moment gave the early Church, as it spread into gentile lands, a clear directive to abandon the laws pertaining to diet as well as the many other folkways which had become Jewish law over the centuries. Christianity's concern with diet became one with its spiritual practice: fasting, abstinence, and that sacred meal in which the basic necessities of life, simple food and drink, become the essence, the body and blood of the Master—the meal of thanksgiving or eucharist.

In considering what was eaten by the people of biblical times it must be borne in mind that the diet really did not change appreciably once the People of Israel settled the Promised Land. Therefore, the Old Testament references to diet hold for New Testament times as well, at least among the common folk. The wealthy of any civilization eat differently from the have-nots, usually more chaotically due to the ability to afford foods grown long distances away, a greater amount of what are considered delicacies, and more expensive foods in general, especially meat. In 1 Kings 4:23 we find a list of King Solomon's provisions for one day: "ten fat oxen and twenty pasture-fed cattle, a hundred sheep, besides harts, gazelles, roebucks, and fatted fowl." All this is not to say that he was not a grain eater. The list includes one hundred fifty five bushels of fine flour (ground from only the inner kernel of wheat and without the bran) and three hundred sixty bushels of meal (whole wheat flour). Given the probability of exaggeration, the list demonstrates a high meat consumption for the royal family household, attending decision makers, and advisors. The prophet Amos denounces the wealthy who "eat lambs from the flock and calves from the midst of the stall," (Amos 6:4). Perhaps this is why although the common people may be rather balanced and freedom loving, those in power may be war-like and make the decisions which require the common people to fight their battles for them. Except where specifically noted, biblical references are to commonly consumed food.

Ecclesiasticus 39:26 states, "The chief necessities of human life are water, fire, iron, and salt, flour, honey, and milk, the juice of the grape, oil and clothing." There is no mention of meat here, because in biblical times meat was not a regular part of the diet but reserved for religious festivals such as the Passover (Exodus 12:21, 24; Mark 14:12). This celebration food was also used for entertaining an honored guest as it is reported Abraham did in taking a calf from the herd when three strangers arrived (Genesis 18:7), community celebrations such as marriage feasts where both oxen and fat calves are mentioned (Matthew 22:4), or special moments of family celebration as in the return of the prodigal, "Bring the fatted calf and kill it, and let us eat and make merry," (Luke 15:23). Perhaps, a clue to meat used for a lesser celebration is given by the brother of the prodigal who laments, "You know how I have slaved for you all these years; I never once disobeyed your orders; and you never gave me so much as a kid for a feast with my friends." So it can be said that meat was eaten, although not with great regularity, and was a food used at times of special celebration. Meat and animal products were not the staple food of these people. When the great famine occurred, which resulted in the patriarch Joseph being reunited with his family, it was grain which was bought for food. Genesis 47:14 states, "Joseph gathered up all the money that was found in the land of Egypt and in the land of Canaan for the grain which they bought . . . " Then the "Egyptians came to Joseph and said, 'Give us food; why should we die before your eyes? For our money is gone.' And Joseph answered, 'Give your cattle, and I will give you food in exchange for your cattle, if your money is gone,' " (Genesis 47:15b–16). Later, they sell themselves into slavery and their land as well. Joseph buys them for Pharoah and says, "Now here is seed for you and you shall sow the land. And at the harvests you shall give a fifth to Pharoah, and four fifths shall be your own as seed for the field and as food for yourselves and your households, and as food for your little ones," (Genesis 47:23, 24). The "flocks and herds," mentioned as traded for grain in verse 17, evidently were not considered food for everyday sustenance.

Flesh eating in general was widespread with fish being the most commonly consumed animal quality food. The Children of Israel complained bitterly about their diet to Moses as he led them across the wilderness to the promised land, and that complaint gives us a clue to the nature of their diet in Egypt, "We remember the fish we ate in Egypt for nothing, the cucumbers, the melons, the leeks, the onions and the garlic," (Numbers 11:5). This is not to say that their diet was devoid of grain, usually eaten as bread, for we hear their complaint again mentioning this bread in conjunction with a description of one of the common methods of cooking meat, namely boiling: "Would that we had died by the hand of the Lord in the land of Egypt, when we sat by the fleshpots and ate bread to the full; for you have brought this whole assembly out into this wilderness to kill us with hunger," (Exodus 16:3). On that forty year journey, food was provided from "heaven" in the form of manna and quail. The former has been explained by scholars as possibly a form of lichen which blew off the cliffs on which it grew and was found usable by beating it into a flour and cooking with it. Whatever manna actually was, it was reminiscent of bread enough to be designated "bread from heaven" by the writer of Exodus, a name picked up by the writer of the Gospel of John ascribing that same name to Jesus (6:31–35, 49–51). Quail also "covered the camp" and provided food. The death of thousands of birds has been recorded many times in recent history caused by temperature inversions which cause whole flocks of heat sensitive birds to crash to their deaths, littering the ground with their carcasses. There were no domesticated fowl in Israel at the time of Elijah (850 B.C.), but by the time of Jesus fowl must have been plentiful since Jesus uses the simile of the mother hen taking her brood under her wing (Matthew 23:37), and it was a rooster crowing which reminded Peter of the accuracy of his master's prediction of denial (Mark 14:72).

There is no mention of hen's eggs in the Old Testament, although wild bird's eggs may have well have been eaten, assuming that the gathering of them as reported in Isaiah 10:14 was for that purpose. By Jesus' time eggs were eaten, and the description of a father giving his son the food asked for in Luke 11:11, 12, gives us another clue to food consumed. Those verses are rendered in the King James Version: "If a son shall ask bread of any of you that is a father, will he give him a stone? Or if he ask a fish, will he for a fish give him a serpent? Or if he shall ask an egg, will he offer him a scorpion?" Jesus goes on to say that if earthly fathers know how to give good gifts to their children, surely the father of all will give the Holy Spirit to those who ask him. The connection between bread and stone, fish and serpent, egg and scorpion is one of shape. It would be possible to fool a child momentarily giving a slightly rounded brown stone the shape of a loaf of bread, or a snake instead of a small fish, or a scorpion curled up in a ball, as they do when picked up, instead of an egg. At the feeding of the five thousand Jesus accomplishes the miracle with barley loaves and fish, (Matthew 14: 17), evidently the food which was most available. Bread, fish, and, occasionally, eggs were a part of the diet of Jesus' day.

Fruit was eaten in season, dried, or pressed as wine and olive oil. The favorite fruit eaten fresh appears to be figs, especially the first ones of the year, the Hebrew word for which actually means "first born." Isaiah 28: 4 tells how irresistable these delicacies were: "When a man sees it, he eats it up as soon as it is in his hand." Jesus, looking for a fig to eat and finding none on the tree curses the tree and it dies, (Matthew 21: 19). Although it is difficult to know exactly what is meant, the word "apple" is used to designate some similar fruit. Pomegranates and the date palm are also mentioned. However, olives, grapes, and figs are the dominant fruit, with the first two being used for oil and wine, the latter being the most commonly consumed whole fruit, often dried in cakes to take on one's travels as described in 1 Samuel 25: 18; 30: 12.

Vegetables were not grown in any great variety if we are to depend upon biblical reference to inform us. Onions and leeks were cultivated widely and cucumbers are mentioned only in Isaiah and Jeremiah besides being included in the list of complaints by the Children of Israel mentioned above. The vegetable which dominates biblical writing and serves as the principle food is grain, and it is consumed usually as bread. It is the solid food mentioned as one of the three gifts from God by the psalmist in Psalm 104:15, "wine to gladden the heart, oil to make his face shine, and bread to strengthen man's heart." Bread is the food mentioned as the basic, daily form of sustenance asked for in the Lord's prayer. In fact, the expression "eat bread and drink water" could be used to signify eating and drinking in general, (1 Kings 13:8, 9; 16–19). The same is true of Greek where to eat bread equals to take a meal. The same is also true for English where *meal* means whatever is eaten at *meal*time—today decreasingly whole ground grain or meal. Being so basic to life, bread is also an appropriate offering to the gods in all of the ancient Near East. It is mentioned in Babylonian and Mesopotamian ritual, and David's eating the "showbread" or "bread of the Presence" in 1 Samuel 21:6, is referred to by Jesus in Mark 2:26, as an example of precedence in his claim that religion was made for its adherants, not the adherants for the religion.

Bread was baked in three ways. First, on hot, flat stones on which a fire had been built then raked away. The dough was placed on the stone, then covered over with the ashes. The bread Elijah found in 1 Kings 19:6, was cooked this way. A griddle or flat earthenware, later iron, dish was also used. If those used were like those found at the archaeological dig at Tell ed-Duweir the loaves would have been flat and about eighteen inches in diameter. Ovens were the most widely used method in more recent biblical times and took the form of large, inverted earthenware jars under which fires were built. The bread was baked on the stones lining the bottoms of the oven. Large cylinders of earthenware may also have been used and the dough pressed onto the hot interior or exterior walls. That method is in use today in Arab countries and is also a common way of cooking chappatis in India. These techniques produced round loaves like the pita or Syrian bread for sale in American super markets. The Hebrew word for "cake" comes from a root meaning "round," and one of Gideon's soldiers, in Judges 7:13, dreams that a barley loaf rolls into the Midianite camp.

Grain was also eaten by rolling it between one's palms to husk it and then consumed raw as a "trail mix" readily available in a country abounding in grain fields and scattered stands planted by birds. Jesus' disciples were called to task by the Pharisees over just such an action when they did it on the Sabbath. This precipitated the exchange ending with Jesus' citing King David's eating the bread of the Presence. Although this is not the preferred method for eating grain, it is tasty as a snack as I found out one year when our green manure crop of rye was not all turned under, and it set seed.

We can also expect that a kind of gruel or porridge was made as is found in all grain eating cultures, and that barley, especially, would have been added to soups and stews, as it is today even by the commercial canned soup manufacturers.

Parching or roasting represents an often mentioned method of cooking grain and is one of the foods offered to Ruth by Boaz in a description of the kind of meal eaten at noon in the midst heavy field work, " 'Come here, and eat some bread and dip your morsel in the wine.' So she sat beside the reapers, and he passed to her parched grain; and she ate until she was satisfied, and she had some left over," (Ruth 2: 14).

Wheat and barley were the primary grains, but millet and spelt were used in bread, as the interesting recipe in Ezekiel 4: 9 recommends: "And you take wheat and barley, beans and lentils, millet and spelt, and put them into a single vessel, and make bread of them." This recipe does not produce a fluffy, white bread, nor does it produce a lack of fiber in the diet, nor does it produce an elderly population consuming a patent concoction of processed psillium seeds and sugar "for regularity." This bread is a meal. It combines the complementary proteins of beans and grains, ample complex carbohydrates to be broken down slowly into energy-giving sugars, necessary fats and oils, and the minerals of the soils in which its ingredients were grown. There are no animal waste products trapped in flesh, no endocrine levels appropriate to a creature terrified by impending death. The recipe is very much akin to the "grain bread" recipes we find in macrobiotic cookbooks. Upon eating bread made from a grain bread recipe one understands how prisoners in the past were able to maintain life on bread and water.

Condiments were used to add flavor to this simple food, and we find mention of mint, rue, dill, cumin, mustard, coriander, capers, saffron, and cinnamon. Honey was sometimes available and highly prized. The promised land was anticipated as a land flowing with "milk and honey" (Exodus 3:8). This special food tastes tremendously sweet to the palate unaccustomed to refined cane sugar and is, therefore, the prime simile for sweetness in the Bible (Judges 14:8; Psalm 119:103; Ezekiel 3:3; Revelation 10:9). The writer of Proverbs 25:25 recognized the danger of consuming too much of this intense food, though, and admonishes his readers, "It is not good to eat too much honey, so be sparing of complimentary words." We are called by this advice to be careful with compliments lest we seem obsequious and weak, just as the over consumption of honey leaves one with an eventual sugar low, flaccid and weak.

Beverages were primarily wine, water, and milk, although it would be difficult to imagine that with honey, mint, cinnamon, and aromatic wild plants available some form of tea was not also drunk. A spiced wine is offered to Jesus at the crucifixion (Mark 15:23). Wine was drunk at mealtime mixed with water, a tradition which still holds in the preparation of the wine at Christian eucharistic celebrations, although adding water to the wine has come to be seen as a symbolic representation of the description that both water and blood flowed from Jesus' side when he was lanced to assure his death.

Milk was drunk mixed with water, and first century A.D. Roman writing mentions the use of camel's milk in this fashion mixed three parts water to one part milk. The first century B.C. Roman poet Virgil in his agricultural poems, *The Georgics,* makes it clear that the milk of goats and ewes is preferred and describes methods for increasing goat's milk production in Book 3, lines 393 to 397. He mentions the interesting custom of the nomads of Rhodope and the Getic wilderness mixing fresh horse's blood with sheep's milk in order to curdle it, (Book 3, Lines 460 to 463). Cow's milk should be reserved for calves:

> Nor will your cows, as in our fathers' day,
> When newly calved fill pails with snowy milk,
> But save their udders for their cherished offspring.[10]

In trying to change the dietary habits of their "fathers' day," and get people off cow's milk, Virgil sounds a great deal like a modern day macrobiotic. Goat's milk was the norm in his day and is the recommendation of macrobiotics for those who feel they must drink milk. Virgil was not flying in the face of a Roman Dairy Council whose nutritional research "proved" that adults cannot consider their diets adequate without cow's milk and whose advertizing and lobbying promoted the same end. As with the Romans, it was goat's milk which was the most commonly used as a beverage by biblical people, with some sage advice being offered by the writer of Proverbs: "When the grass is gone, and the new growth appears, and the herbage of the mountains is gathered, the lambs will provide your clothing, and the goats the price of a field; there will be enough goat's milk for your food, for the food of your household and maintenance for your maidens" (Proverbs 27:27). We find here that sheep are primarily for clothing, and goats for milk and for bartering in purchasing a more necessary commodity—land. The land would be used for growing principle foods. Usually milk was made into cheese and curds which kept better in the hot climate and were far more beneficial in their partially digested state. Mother's milk was and still is considered the appropriate food for infants, and there are several references to breast feeding (Isaiah 28:9; 60:16; Job 24:9; Psalm 22:9, and others).

That basic human necessity, salt, is referred to many times in the Bible. Dr. Ishizuka considered its balance with potassium to be necessary for good health. The potassium/sodium balance is recognized by modern medicine as well with great concern being given to electrolyte levels and attention to the diets of those with heart disease, usually the result of a yang diet high in salt. Many patients suffering heart attacks are put on a potassium intravenous feeding immediately under the assumption that sodium levels are relatively too high. Salt is on the list of necessities of life cited above in Ecclesiasticus (39:26). Job asks, "Can that which is tasteless be eaten without salt?" Covenants were sealed by eating salt with someone, making the agreement permanent. Reference to this is found in Ezra 4:14 where parties were bound to the king by virtue of having eaten the palace salt. "Covenant of salt" is an expression found in Numbers 18:19, and Second Chronicles 13:5. In Mark 9:50, Jesus commands, "Have salt in yourselves and be at peace with one another." This statement refers to the covenant, and graciousness to one another is also reflected in Paul's advice to the Colossians, "Let your speech always be gracious, seasoned with salt, so that you may know how you ought to answer everyone." (Colossians 4:6). Jesus calls his disciples the "salt of the earth," (Matthew 5:13) in reference to the life-giving and purifying qualities of salt. It is the same as saying, "You are basic, you are necessary." Salt was used in temple worship both mixed with incense and spread on sacrificial animals. Although much could be made of Lot's wife turning to a pillar of salt when she looked back, it is thought that the story is part of folk legend to explain an unusual rock salt pillar in the region of the Dead Sea.

As might be expected from Dr. Ishizuka's discovery of the potassium/sodium balance and George Ohsawa's recognition that in these elements are represented the predominance of either the expansive or contractive forces of the universe, the correct use of salt is a primary concern in macrobiotics. This concern extends to the quality of the salt used and that it be a naturally produced sea salt, not a "refined" salt with aluminium silicate, sugar, and iodine added (only one of a number of elements naturally present in sea salt). The dominant taste in macrobiotic food should be sweet. The sweetness inherant in grains, fruits and vegetables can be enhanced by the judicious use of salt. If food tastes salty at all there is too much salt being used. Perhaps this was Job's recognition in his asking how tasteless food could be made tasty without salt. This compound of the element sodium is, indeed, a necessity whose use in proper proportion allows our whole physiology to remain in balance without stress.

There is really remarkable correspondance between the diet of these peoples and the macrobiotic dietary recommendations for those living in similar latitude and climate. In the predominance of grains and legumes, the consumption of locally grown fruits and vegetables in season, the variety in cooking techniques, the periodic use of animal flesh, especially fish, commensurate with the nutritional demands of a rugged life style, even in the use of goat's milk over that of bovines, we find reflected in the pages of the Bible the dietary pattern typical of ancient cultural tradition.

It is the understanding in macrobiotics that this diet is most basic and true to the needs of human beings. It has a grounding effect on those who practice it, keeping them in touch with cultural and intuitional roots which reach far back into the history of the human species. Those early peoples of Wadi Kubbaniya knew the times and the seasons; they moved with the grace of grain in the wind. The people of the Bible, whose faith led them into the unknown, knew that a bountiful universe would provide as the changing seasons required. Their diet was dominated by the vegetables which sprang up under the rain, flourished only where appropriate, responded to the farmer's care, and adapted as necessary to changing conditions. These people knew well the truth which Paul proclaims to the Church in Corinth, ". . . you are God's garden," (1 Corinthians 1:9), that we, too, are being cultivated, planted, weeded, watered, and tilled, deep in our being by a caring gardener. We are called to accept the rain and sun, the weeding and the planting as does the garden whose produce we consume, and we, too, will bear good fruit.

There are several interesting references to food in the Bible which bear on this discussion and provide us with some insight into dietary philosophy and customs. One concern the importance of diet and fertility. At a time when upward of twenty percent of American couples are infertile, some advice in this direction is appropriate. Samson's mother is visited by an angel and told, ". . . Drink no wine or strong drink and eat nothing unclean, for lo you shall conceive and bear a son," (Judges 13:4, 5). The advice is repeated in verses 7, and 13–15 with the latter verses also adding "anything which comes from the vine" to the prohibitions. Manoah, Samson's mother offers grain and a goat to God in thanksgiving for the visitation of the angel. She *does* conceive and gives birth to one of the strongmen of all time. The most important part of this advice may well be that there was awareness on the part of the writer of Judges that, indeed, diet and fertility are related. Recent scientific work has born out the accuracy of the angel's advice. For instance, alcohol is known to affect fertility and the size of the newborn. It must be remembered that the advice is not very extensive, just a small adjustment, because the balance of Manoah's diet was whole grains, beans, and fresh vegetables, organically grown and locally produced.

Another story deals with the effect of food on appearance, intellectual ability and intuitive faculties. Daniel, chapter 1:3–20, relates a story of King Nebuchadnezzar of Babylon's desire to have some of the new captives from Israel serve in the palace. He sends his chief eunuch to gather some young people from the royal families and nobility captured in the 598 B.C. seige of Jerusalem. Among those selected were Daniel, Shadrach, Meshach, and Abednego. The orders were to have those selected fed well with the usual palace food which, as noted above, was not what the common person ate, but richer and far more chaotic. Daniel refused to eat the food and asked that he and his three companions be given ". . . vegetables to eat and water to drink," (Daniel 1:12) for ten days as a test. The eunuch was afraid that they would waste away and that he would receive the king's wrath for not feeding them properly, but he is convinced on the basis of trying it as a test. We are told, "At the end of ten days it was seen that they were better in appearance and fatter in flesh than all the youths who ate the king's rich food. So the steward took away their rich food and the wine they were to drink and gave them vegetables," (Daniel 1: 15, 16). The king found these four to be "ten times better" than his own magicians, enchanters, and wise men. There may well have been some hesitation to consume the king's "rich food" because it did not follow the guidelines set down for the Hebrew people in their law, but the story also shows that, even among the "royalty and nobility" of the Hebrew people there was a simpler food consumed than that at the court of Nebuchadnezzar. "The king's food," it could be argued, might just produce the kind of mentality which would want to lay seize to Jerusalem. In any case, food, appearance, intuitive and intellectual ability are linked here, twenty five hundred years before we had to be advised, "you are what you eat."

Christianity was not an ethnic religion but spread to the whole Mediterranean world within twenty years of Jesus' death and resurrection. Had the Jerusalem element within the movement prevailed and required all Christians first to observe Jewish initiation rites and customs, the Hebrew dietary code might well be observed by Christians. Peter's vision of Acts 10: 11, in which Peter is told that God has cleansed those foods named unclean by the dietary code, was required because such a code was inappropriate in the face of such rapid expansion to varied climates and cultures, nor would the diet of Palestine have been appropriate for the early Christian inhabitants of the more yin, colder, climate, for instance, of what are now the British Isles. We do not find specific dietary guidelines in Christianity except for certain days when meat is abstained from and times when fasting is recommended.

The only specific mention of Jesus' fasting is as preparation for his baptism by John in the Jordan and by inference in such teaching as Mark 9: 29. Jesus is quoted as saying that some kinds of exorcism require prayer and fasting. The assumption must be that he prayed and fasted in order to accomplish such a healing. However, not all manuscripts include the word "fasting." His style was feasting, not fasting, and he expected his disciples to follow his lead. He is quoted to that effect in Matthew 9: 14–15, "Then John's disciples came to him with the question: 'Why do we and the Pharisees fast, but your disciples do not?' Jesus replied, 'Can you expect the bridegroom's friends to go mourning while the bridegroom is with them? The time will come when the bridegroom will be taken away from them; that will be the time for them to fast.' " Even if this quotation is an interpolation of the early church, it must represent the case that there was no fasting while Jesus was with them but that fasting was observed in the post resurrection community. There were times of fasting in the early church as recorded in Acts 13:2–3; 14:23, and mention of fasting in preparation for baptism in the church of the late second century appears in the writing of Tertullian. This approach to diet and spirituality was elaborated upon over the years to the point where fasting was required before receiving communion, and abstinence from meat demanded on Wednesdays, Fridays, and Lent. Some adjustments have been made in these disciplines, but the church, to this day, recognizes the purifying power of fasting as a dietary discipline.

Christianity is a catholic or universal religion. The word catholic comes from a contraction of the Greek *kata* and *holou* which really means according to the whole. Not being limited, historically, to a certain people or place, dietary guidelines could not be drawn. But, of all the religions of the world, there is none in which eating plays a more prominent role. The prominence of the sacred meal, the central act of Christian worship, is faithful to the style of the master Jesus and was instituted by him at "the last supper" as the act, which would call forth his presence in the midst of his followers. Jesus describes himself as one who "came eating and drinking" (Luke 7:34a) in contradistinction to John the Baptizer whose chief characteristic was his asceticism. What was characteristic of Jesus is that his style so centered around table fellowship that, in verse 34b, he quotes the Pharisees and lawyers as saying, "Look at him! a glutton and a drinker, a friend of tax gatherers and sinners." His willingness to eat with social outcasts was one of the main causes of the aggravation of the Pharisees and religious authorities.[11] However, it was one of the main characteristics of his mode of expressing his conviction that the kingdom of God had dawned.

Jesus ate with all who invited him; we do not hear of his having turned an invitation down. He attended wedding feasts such as that in Cana, spent time in the homes of his disciples and friends, stayed with friends like Lazarus, Mary, and Martha in Bethany when in the Jerusalem area. He was no reclusive ascetic. He even invited himself to someone's house on occasion. Luke recounts the story of Zacchaeus, the superintendent of taxes in Jericho who was so short in stature that he had to climb a tree to see Jesus. When Jesus came by he was evidently so taken by the zeal of this little man that he said, "Zacchaeus, be quick and come down; I must come and stay with you today," (Luke 19:5). The report goes on to recount, "There was a general murmur of disapproval. 'He has gone in,' they said, 'to be the guest of a sinner,' " (Luke 19:7). Yet, he recognized the need for balance which is satisfied by times alone in prayer. Jesus' prime teaching on prayer, The Lord's Prayer, is acknowledged by scholars to be a table prayer. The story of the anointing of Jesus with precious oil told in Luke 7:36–50, takes place in the setting of his being a dinner guest of a Pharisee. Is it any wonder that this theme of feasting and table fellowship, given the impetus of the command, "Do this in remembrance of me," at the last supper, continues to be the principle act of Christian worship? Tertullian, writing toward the end of the second Century reports,

> The Sacrament of the Eucharist, which was instituted by the Lord at mealtime and enjoined upon all, we take in assemblies before daybreak. . . ."[12]

The church has remained true to its predecessors of the Apostolic age who ". . . devoted themselves to the apostles' teaching and fellowship, to the breaking of bread and the prayers," (Acts 2:42). James Breech, the Canadian scholar even goes so far as to state,

> One of the primary ways in which they attempted to continue living in the dimension which Jesus had revealed was through the early Christian practice of engaging in communal meals, enacted in memory of Jesus' table fellowship. This is where the continuity between Jesus and early Christianity is to be found.[13]

So intertwined is the meaning of joy, celebration and food that the word "feast" means both the event and the activity engaged in to celebrate the event. Unless designated "fast days" the festivals of the liturgical year are called "feasts." Just as at the first American Thanksgiving, the meal is celebrated in honor of the day and as an outer expression of an inner attitude of thanksgiving for abundance. In the Christian Eucharist the abundant presence of the master in the midst of those so celebrating through simple food and drink makes Christianity a religion of table fellowship like no other.

The concern of macrobiotics with the quality of food which is eaten speaks to a theology which recognizes that the body is a temple of the Holy Spirit: "Do you not know that your body is a shrine of the indwelling Holy Spirit, and the Spirit is God's gift to you? You do not belong to yourselves; you were bought at a price. Then honor God in your body," (1 Corinthians 6: 19, 20). Such belief springs naturally from the central doctrine of Christianity, the incarnation. When this belief, that the creator of all was manifest totally in the body of Jesus, is joined with Paul's theology of total union of believers with Jesus (celebrated in baptism) the result is the understanding that the body is not simply the repository of the spiritual principle but, while alive, of cosmic significance. It is to be treated with the respect due any holy place. This also means active concern for the natural, social, and political environment in which the body dwells as well as a willingness to oppose those who would manipulate and destroy human life in any way. As Raimundo Panikkar, Professor of Comparative Religions at the University of California, states, "saving the body, in this way, cannot be separated from saving the soul."[14]

Christianity's table orientation is not limited to this life. The consummation of all activity in the universe is symbolized in the heavenly banquet where the unity which results from sitting at table together finds its home in the world to come, when all nations will be of one blood and partake of one, holy food. That promise and vision is realized in the awareness of the sacredness of every meal, the necessity for a moment of thanksgiving or blessing. The realization that as above so below makes every meal a reflection of the endless heavenly banquet. In the simple and pure food we consume is found the Lord of life and from it is built his temple. In table fellowship over lovingly prepared, whole and holy food, we can say with the psalmist, "O taste and see that the Lord is good!" (Psalm 34:8a).

---

[1] Aihara, *Seven Basic Macrobiotic Principles,* p. 5.
[2] for a list of the 12 Laws of Change see Kushi, *The Book of Macrobiotics,* pp. 7ff.
[3] *Science 82,* November issue, p. 73.
[4] Leon-Portilla, *Native MesoAmerican Spirituality,* p. 215.
[5] Ibid. p. 198 ff.
[6] Tooker, *Native North American Spirituality of The Eastern Woodlands,* p. 62, ff.
[7] Josephus, *The Works of Flavius Josephus,* p. 675.
[8] Ibid. p. 674.
[9] Kushi, *The Book of Macrobiotics,* p. 66.
[10] Wilkinson, L. P., *Virgil, The Georgics,* Book 3, Lines 177–179.
[11] see Breech, *The Silence of Jesus,* Chapter 5, for a full and interesting discussion of this interpretation.
[12] Bettenson, *Documents of the Christian Church,* p. 107.
[13] Breech, *The Silence of Jesus,* p. 59.
[14] *Epiphany,* Vol. 3, No. 4, p. 31.

Chapter 9

Gratitude

"Give thanks whatever happens."
(First Thessalonians 5 : 18)

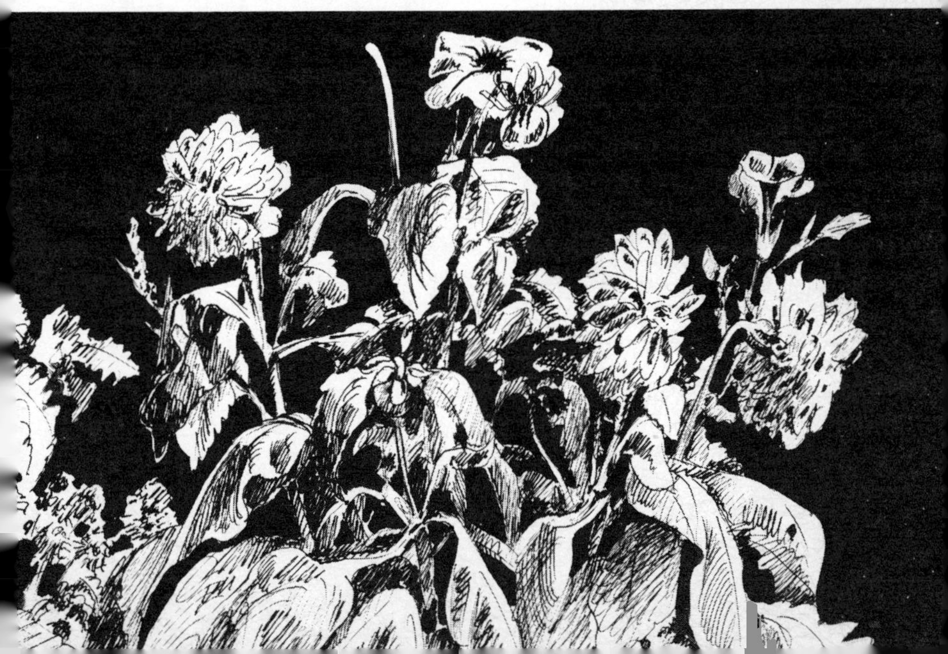

THE THREE-YEAR OLD TOOK THE LITTLE PRESENT with some embarrassment, turned and ran into another room. His mother called him back and when he returned obediently she said, "Aunt Betty gave you a pretty present; what do you say?"

How many times have we heard that same question during our own upbringing? Each of us has been prompted by various adults during our growing years to make the simple expression of gratitude: "Thank you!" What is it which prompts East and West to hold gratitude as both appropriate and necessary? What does this near universal expression do for both the giver and the thanks-giver?

There are cultures and religions in which we find no specific expression of gratitude. The Australian aborigine demonstrates no excessive expression of appreciation or gratitude, and that fact has been interpreted adversely by some. Giving is such a fixed habit in aboriginal society that gratitude does not seem to be expected. The interchange which occurs with constant giving and receiving is an outer demonstration of the inner truth that everything is a differentiation of one infinity. In a universe created from one great "giver of every good and perfect gift," (James 1:17) the sense of cosmos should be all that is necessary. After all, who is there to thank if creation is one? Rather than being a shortcoming, lack of expressions of gratitude may be a demonstration that the apparently ungrateful are actually more highly evolved than those of us who have forgotten that we partake of infinity.

Lack of expressed gratitude may also be the result of a belief that all that happens follows inexorable laws of cause and effect, a sort of Newtonian mechanics theology in which one thing follows another with no possibility for spontaneous manifestation. Such an understanding tends to follow a theology of predestination or of karma. The Jain returns no thanks for answered prayer, for sins forgiven, for hopes fulfilled. Everything which happens to him in this life is in direct payment for his own good actions in past existence. But such an understanding also reflects the belief that the universe is not two, and that whatever we do has its effect either now or later. Everything is interdependent, interrelated, woof and warp of the same cosmic tapestry.

There is little room for gratitude in determinism. The mechanical procession of events in the life of a fatalist gives no cause for a heartfelt thank you. It would be like thanking water for running downhill. Among the fatalistic Egyptians gratitude is said to be almost unknown. In fact, there is no exact phrase for "thank you" in the old Egyptian language. In Coptic, "I am grateful" is rendered "a favor has been received." This contrasts markedly with biblical injunctions to "make thanksgiving your sacrifice to God and make good your vows to the most high" (Psalm 50: 14) or ". . . give thanks every day for everything to our God and Father," (Ephesians 5: 20).

The biblical view reflects the belief that all we are and all we have is a gift from a loving God. Perhaps it is in this that we seem to see the greatest disparity between the theology implied in macrobiotic philosophy and the Judeo-Christian belief. The latter belief is personal not only in the manifestation of the divine within the depths of each person but in the very nature of that divinity, the "one infinity" posited by macrobiotic philosophy. "One infinity" is the term used in macrobiotics for the "one God and Father of all, who is over all and through all and in all," (Ephesians 4: 6). True to the Eastern heritage of macrobiotic philosophy the "one infinity" is not portrayed as personal, yet this vivifying energy is certainly seen as an appropriate recipient of our thanksgiving. The writings of George Ohsawa and each of his students are filled with admonitions to give thanks and to adopt an attitude of gratefulness. In *The Book of Macrobiotics*, Chapter 4, Michio Kushi suggests that we give thanks for the food we eat and the utensils used in the meal (p. 78); that every morning and evening we set aside time to offer our gratitude to our ancesters (p. 83); that "principles for human relations with neighboring people as well as with people who are living at a distance include: a "Spirit of gratitude for whatever we receive, material and spiritual . . ." (p. 93). This spirit is also to include ". . . our gratitude for mountains and rivers, land and ocean, trees and flowers, birds and fishes, animals and vegetables, the sky and the stars" (p. 93). The final principle offered in a list of six "principles of our macrobiotic way of life" is: "Be grateful for difficulties." (p. 97). This injunction is consonant with biblical understanding. Surely one would be grateful for those events in which God is perceived as acting, and Job, that sometimes patient man of difficulty, was advised by his friend, Elihu: "He delivers the afflicted by their affliction, and opens their ear by adversity," (Job 36: 15). Herman Aihara even defines macrobiotics within the context of engendering gratitude:

> Macrobiotics is an attempt to experience and express gratitude towards everything, beginning with a grain of rice, a bowl of soup or a piece of bread. It teaches us to appreciate everything, without exception, including pain, disease, hatred, and intolerance.[1]

Such a profusion of suggestions for gratitude should advise the Western student of macrobiotics that perhaps the impersonal designation of the divinity as "one infinity" is impersonal in name only. The life of the divine, found as it is in all manifestation as well as beyond all manifestation gives occasion for thanksgiving to and for even those things which, by Western reckoning, are considered inanimate. That love which George Ohsawa describes as so vast as to make even antagonisms complementary flows from a source to which our gratitude may be directed. Neither macrobiotic nor believer in Judeo-Christian theology need fear the fate of the atheist described by Dante Gabriel Rosetti,

> The worst moment for the atheist is when he is really thankful and has nobody to thank.[2]

Sometimes the virtually worldwide custom of giving thanks before meals is initiated with the words, "Let us return thanks." The giving of thanks is, truly, our return gift, an expression from our heart to the heart of all, an interplay of yin and yang, a celebration of unity. Without the conscious expression of gratitude nothing is offered to balance the gift from the source of all consciousness. We become unbalanced; our lack of giving heartfelt thanks, in accordance with the law that we reap what we sow, eventually results in the diminution of those gifts we recognize as "good and perfect." We begin to reap a meager harvest:

> Remember: sparse sowing, sparse reaping; sow bountifully, and you will reap bountifully . . . God loves a cheerful giver. And it is in God's power to provide you richly with every good gift; thus you will have ample means within yourself to meet every situation, with enough and to spare for every good cause . . . Now he who provides seed for sowing and bread for food will provide the seed for you to show; he will multiply it and swell the harvest of your benevolence, and you will always be rich enough to be generous. Through our action such generosity will issue in thanksgiving to God, for as a piece of willing service this is not only a contribution towards the needs of God's people; more than that, it overflows in a flood of thanksgiving to God. (2 Corinthians 9:6–12)

Pindar, the lyric poet of fifth Century B.C. Greece, describes the results of ingratitude by the fate of Ixion, a signal ingrate. Bound by the command of the gods to his winged wheel Ixion declares to all that one should repay the benefactor with kindly recompense. The results of ingratitude are described in Greek legend as well in the story of Atalante and Melanion. Melanion won Atalante, beating her in a footrace by dropping golden apples of Aphrodite which Atalante stopped to pick up. They were wed and went to Boiota, but their happiness was short-lived. Melanion had forgotten to thank Aphrodite for her help. As they rested in a grotto near the temple of Kybele, the goddess threw a spell upon them turning them to lions forbidden to know the joys of mutual love.

The necessary balance achieved by giving, as well as the increased receiving which accompanies generosity, make the act of giving a blessed one in the teachings of Jesus, "It is more blessed to give than to receive," (Acts 20:35). This act of giving thanks may, be more than a verbal one, and may issue from deeds of benevolence, as Paul suggests above.

Such an understanding has resulted in the formation of the society of Hōtoku, organized by the disciples of Ninomiya Sontoku, the peasant sage of Japan, (1787–1856). This wise man's teaching was centered in the idea of gratitude to heaven and earth and man for blessings received: to heaven for the light of the sun and moon, for growth and decay; to earth for the trees, grain, birds, animals and fish; to man for his various offices and labors. Hence, the first principle of conduct is *to make suitable return* for these blessings. The manner in which such return can be made is set forth in Ninomiya's teaching, known as *Hōtoku.* Members of the society are, by their conduct, to show gratitude for all the blessings they have received, to be industrious, and to live so within their income that there will be a surplus which may be used to improve the environment.

George Ohsawa makes the same point within a discussion of good humor as an indicator of good health:

> In the Occident one says, "Give and take;" in the East we say, "Give, give and give infinitely." You lose nothing at all by imitating us for you have received life itself—the whole universe—without paying. You are the unique son or daughter of the Infinite Universe; it creates, animates, destroys and reproduces everything necessary for you. If you know this everything will come to you in abundance.[3]

In macrobiotic philosophy the rationale for the necessity of giving is found in the context of the spiral of manifestation. This spiral is described as originating with the undifferentiated One and spiraling inward through seven successive levels of manifestation: polarization (yin/yang), vibration, preatomic particles, elements, vegetable life, animal life, human life. This is the yang or contractive, ever-tightening sequence.[4] From the point of human life the spiral then expands outward, unwinding back toward the infinite One through the non-physical worlds, astral, spiritual and divine, recognized in seven ascending levels of judgment—physical, sensory, sentimental, intellectual, social, ideological, supreme.[5] In a March, 1975, lecture, Michio Kushi describes the connection between the spirals of physicalization and divinization:

> The spiritual world, the world of our developing judgment, is the world of expansion. The world of physicalization is the world of contraction. So, at the stage of existence we are at now, it is much better to give out, give out, give out. This giving out helps us, as we beome more highly developed, to also become lighter and lighter until, at last, we reach supreme judgment. Now, if we receive something, and then we give that away, we have not become lighter. We have only maintained our present condition. In order to become lighter we have to give away more than we receive.[6]

In macrobiotic teaching, the concept of gratitude is central to the right use of the evolutionary spirals of creation, because gratitude is giving, balancing, and a completion of the giving, receiving, giving cycle. Gratitude makes the gift-cycle whole. Giving beyond what is received creates a kind of vacuum which draws us higher up the spiral of spiritual evolution. Heartfelt thanksgiving is always giving more than what is received, because in so doing we give more than gift for gift; we give ourselves, truly all we are and all we have.

We are the benefactors of fantastic universal abundance. In just being alive we are part of an enormous ocean of vitality which gives birth to the physical universe and its cycle of change so well demonstrated in the procession of the seasons. Mother nature never stops, never rests, but she gives birth to life and death constantly, creating, renewing, sustaining, bringing new life from death. This good earth gives us air, food, and water for our sustenance and, even in the face of agricultural mismanagement, presently provides an estimated twice as much food as is necessary to sustain the planet's human population.[7] We receive all this, as George Ohsawa says, "without paying." Those words echo these of Isaiah:

> Come, all who are thirsty, come fetch water; come, you who have no food, buy grain and eat; come and buy, not for money, not for a price. Why spend money and get what is not bread, why give the price of your labor and go unsatisfied? Only listen to me and you will have good food to eat, and you will enjoy the fat of the land. (Isaiah 55: 1, 2)

How is this "buying" to take place if no money is used? An answer may be found in the first verse of Isaiah's next chapter: "Keep justice and do righteousness." We find the key in the balance implied in the word "justice," the balance of giving and thanksgiving expressed in the truth of Jesus' teaching,

> . . . give, and gifts will be given to you. Good measure, pressed down, shaken together, and running over will be poured into your lap; for whatever measure you deal out to others will be dealt to you in return. (Luke 6: 38)

Lest thanksgiving, in any form, be construed as restoring balance and making whole (holy), there must be a word of warning. Beware of apparent gratitude which springs from arrogance manifesting as self righteousness or from the desire for consolation. The first is found in Jesus' parable of the Pharisee and the Publican (Luke 18: 9–14). Two men went to the temple to pray and the law abiding, self righteous Pharisee observed the Publican also at prayer and said, "*I thank thee,* O God, that I am not like other men, greedy, dishonest, adulterous; or, for that matter, like this tax gatherer. I fast twice a week; I pay tithes on all that I get." In giving thanks for faithfully keeping the precepts of his belief system in comparison with the tax gatherer, the Pharisee is conscious only of separation and is fostering that illusion. He *is* giving thanks, but by so doing furthers division rather than healing it. In contrast, the tax gatherer says, "O God, have mercy on me, sinner that I am." The concern of the Publican is simply with himself and his own shortcomings. He casts no aspersions on the Pharisee who believes that divine will is kept by observing man-made codes or, in Jesus' words, that "man was made for the Sabbath." The tax gatherer's stance is one of personal responsibility with an implied understanding that if one's own house is set in order the lawful operation of the cosmos will handle the rest. Jesus finishes the parable by referring to the tax gatherer: "It was this man, I tell you, and not the other, who went home acquitted of his sins. For everyone who exalts himself will be humbled; and, whoever humbles himself will be exalted."

The arrogance of thanksgiving as consolation is particularly widespread because it seems so logical. This form of gratitude runs, "I have so much to be thankful for! There are so many in the world worse off than I am. When I see the television pictures of the starving people in Africa it just makes me so thankful that I have more than enough to eat!" This insidious logic requires the suffering of others in order for the thanksgiver to be thankful. In fact, the greater the suffering of others the greater the cause for thanksgiving! The perpetrator of such thoughts requires a course in remedial compassion.

There is something in the quality of receiving which permits a healthy (whole, inclusive) thanksgiving to be offered rather than the exclusive attitude attending the thanksgiving of both the Pharisee and the person seeing self consolation in the difficulties of others. This quality, Jesus tells us, is found in the way a little child receives: "Truly, I say to you, whoever does not receive the kingdom of God like a child shall not enter it," (Mark 10:15). Many times one hears this quotation used to describe why all should become child-like in order to realize the kingdom of God, but the quote specifically says that it is in the way a child *receives* that the kingdom comes. What are the qualities of a child's receiving? There is no advanced planning to be at the right place at the right time so that the gift will be given; there is no calculation of fair market value once the gift is received; there is no thought of "justice" in receiving such a gift—"Did I deserve it? It should have been more valuable given our relationship! It's about time! Oh, you shouldn't have!" When a child receives he simply receives, accepts without overriding cognitive interference, is filled with the joy of pleasant surprise, and it might be added, may well run away without saying, "Thank you!" Expressed gratitude comes with wisdom. But the groundwork for wholehearted gratitude, the giving of self, is laid in the manner of receiving. The shaky foundation of calculation and exclusivity can only support a facade.

The gift which is not calculated as earned or deserved can only be received as a gift rather than as payment in disguise. Once a gift is accepted as gift then the dependency of the receiver upon the giver can be recognized, acknowledged, and the freedom which attends a gift freely given and freely recieved becomes the genesis point for wholehearted gratitude. For gratitude, itself, to be whole it must issue from the whole person, spring from all one's parts. Recognition of the gift as gift is a function of the intellect, acknowledgement is by the will, and the joy accompanying such recognition and acknowledgement wells up from deep in our inner being. Only when our full selves can be given in our gratitude can it be said that the gift was fully appreciated. Only when thanksgiving at the first six levels of judgment is experienced and then moved through can we attain to the fullness of joy which accompanies all manifestations of unity. The circle is complete and it is completely full.

The ancient world, reflected in the writing of the Old Testament, recognized the centrality of gratitude to a wholesome life. The Psalms are primarily songs of thanks, praise to the giver of that thing for which one is thankful. The Hebrew word for psalm means "song of praise." "Thanks" is offered twenty two times in the Book of Psalms, "thanksgiving" is mentioned eight times, and "praise" and its derivatives occur over one hundred sixty times.

Paul's custom of beginning his letters with a salutation involving thanksgiving was not initiated by him but reflected common custom as has been revealed by Egyptian papyri of the period. His salutations include, "Let me begin by thanking my God, through Jesus Christ, for you all . . ." (Romans 1:8); "I am always thanking God for you." (1 Corinthians 1:4) "I thank my God whenever I think of you," (Philippinas 1:3). Similar salutations are found in: Colossians 1:3; 1 Thessalonians 1:2; 2 Thessalonians 1:3; 2 Timothy 1:3, and others. Such a greeting certainly established a spirit of interdependence at the outset. It would be interesting to know when the custom fell into disuse since it would be rather difficult to observe it and then go on to write a "hate letter."

In Romans 1:18–32, Paul points out the folly of those who refuse to render thanks to God. He details the "vileness" of such people who refuse to honor the One from whom all blessings flow and says, "They have made fools of themselves." Perhaps there is no greater admonition to gratitude than the brief phrase in Ephesians 5:20 to ". . . give thanks every day for everything. . . ." The implications of this injunction are enormous. Imagine what it would be like if this advice were followed. It would mean that thanks would be offered for being rushed, being delayed, for bumping your head, hammering your thumb, being given a difficult time by a store clerk, and for the fender-bender in the supermarket parking lot. Thanks at such times would certainly be reckoned foolish by the wisdom of the world. However, the truth of 1 Corinthians 3:18, 19, is recognized far beyond the boundaries of Christianity.

> If there is anyone among you who fancies himself wise—wise, I mean, by the standards of this passing age—he must become a fool to gain true wisdom. For the wisdom of this world is folly in God's sight.

Those in Romans who "made fools of themselves" must have been reckoned such from the level of supreme judgment rather than that of the average person whose level of judgment seldom is reckoned above "sentimental" on the seven level scale.[8] What is the supreme wisdom in giving "thanks every day for everything?" In so doing the thanksgiver is making a moment by moment statement of radical trust in the rightness of all that is; that nothing happens without purpose or by accident; that whatever happens is for one's benefit; that no gift from the infinite and abundant source of our being is earned; that what others might judge punishment is also a gift for our benefit; that everything is interdependent, and therefore, that "of myself I can do nothing" (John 5:30); that all things are possible. The psalmist says, "offer to God a sacrifice of thanksgiving and make good your vows to the most high." This means that in the act of thanksgiving all vows to the infinite are made good. Meister Eckhart put it this way, "If the only prayer you say in your entire life is, 'Thank you,' that would suffice." Brother David Steindl-Rast sums it up in the title of his recent and most excellent book, *Gratefulness, The Heart of Prayer*.

The wisdom of gratitude is also transcultural. A Seneca Thanksgiving Address recorded in upper New York State at the Tonawanda Reservation runs as follows:

> And now we are gathered in a group. And this is what the Sky Dwellers did: They told us that we should always have love, we who move about on the earth. And this will always be first when people come together, the people who move about on the earth. It is the way it begins when two people meet. They first have the obligation to be grateful that they are thinking well. They greet[9] each other, and, after that, they take up the matter with which just they two are concerned. And this is what our Creator did: He decided, "The people moving about on the earth will simply come to express their gratitude." And this is the obligation of those of us who are gathered: that we continue to be grateful.[10]

When admonitions are virtually identical in spirit and arise from widely divergent cultures the evidence that they contain the truth is overwhelming. The Seneca address makes the point that gratitude is established and willed by the Creator; it is, therefore, a quality inherent in supreme judgment. Paul makes the same point in 1 Thessalonians 5: 16–18:

> Be always joyful; pray continually; give thanks whatever happens; for it is what God in Christ wills for you.

These words, penned in the earliest records of the Christian experience, must reflect the life and teaching of Jesus as they were interpreted and lived out by his early followers. That fact is borne out by the gospel records which associate gratitude with Jesus in several ways. Since thanksgiving is a form of prayer and much of Jesus' prayer life was lived out alone, there are only a few records of thanksgiving specifically related to prayer. At the feeding of the multitudes (Mark 8: 6 and parallels), at the last supper (Mark 14: 23 and parallels, and Paul's report of the last supper in 1 Corinthians 11: 24), we find thanksgiving offered as the first act in prayer at meals. This was according to the custom of the day and to be expected, but the power in the gentle simplicity of the act of thanksgiving over simple gifts cannot be overestimated. Thanksgiving, as we have seen, is an acknowledgment of the awareness of unity. Gratitude expressed wholeheartedly also effects the state in which unity is realized. It is both the result of awareness of unity and the act which causes the completion of the circle of freely giving, the perfect circle of infinite unity. What could be more simple, more intuitional, more basic than expressing gratitude to the creative spirit whose sustaining nourishment creates our bodies from the fruits of the earth? No one at the last supper said, "Wait a minute! Before we eat let's have a prayer of thanks." Reports say, "He took bread, gave thanks, and broke it," (Luke 22: 19). When the power of gratitude is even partially comprehended those are seen to be among the most eloquent words ever penned. They describe a spontaneous bursting forth of thanksgiving for the gift of the thanksgiver himself, for each of us is the unique creation of the vital energies we consume. In giving thanks for that which creates us we give thanks for who we are and what we are, the offspring of infinite creativity.

The power generated by the perfection of the last supper thanksgiving is still celebrated by Christian believers who gather to celebrate *eucharistia,* thanksgiving, as the event which invokes and represents all the power of the infinite present at that first feast. The simplicity of the last supper has become overlaid with nearly two thousand years of liturgical tradition and would appear to someone outside the tradition to be a pretty complicated affair, but the simplest of unleavened bread, essentially flour and water baked, still is taken, thanks given, and the bread broken. The creator, manifest in human flesh, is manifest in that which creates human flesh. Communicants who partake of that food are fed with the bread of thanksgiving. What is remembered most about Jesus by the community of his followers is his thanksgiving and the promise that the creator would be in their midst whenever similar thanksgiving was offered. That act of *eucharistia* has become their principle form of the celebration of their faith—a thankful meal together. How macrobiotic!

Jesus also offers a prayer of thanks for an unusual circumstance: that the highly educated were unable to understand those very things which his simple followers could grasp. The occasion is reported in Luke 10:21, at the return of the seventy two who had been sent out to heal the sick and announce the immanence of the kingdom. Jesus rejoices at their success in an ecstatic reaction described by Luke as his having "exulted in the Holy Spirit," (Luke 10 : 21). The word in Greek which is translated "exulted" means "to leap much for joy." The phrase, "exulted in the Holy Spirit," is an unusual one and denotes a rather special state of cosmic consciousness. The result of this state are the words, "I thank thee, father, Lord of heaven and earth, for hiding these things from the learned and wise and revealing them to the simple. Yes, I thank thee, Father, that such was thy choice," (Luke

10 : 21b). In this special state of consciousness his first and last words are those of thanksgiving.

Anyone who deals with a wide variety of people can attest to the regular occurrence of decisions which demonstrate remarkable native wisdom and the power to make edifying choices in the face of tremendous ignorance and innocence. In such people there is no highly trained cognitive faculty to offer logical commentary in the midst of natural spontaneity. Once an authority has been established, they are willing to accept the dictums of that authority as valid without question. If healing is expected without question then healing unquestionably occurs. The seventy two reported, "In your name, Lord, even the devils submit to us," (Luke 10: 17). These emissaries were able to turn back to front in many peoples' physical condition because of their simple trust. As history has shown, however, the same blind acceptance has meant allowing genocide and permitting societal institutions to commit acts sprung from the dark side of human nature. If the action springs from acceptance of the teachings of a fully conscious being that is one thing, but *non credo* still guarantees full personal responsibility for one's actions in a world populated by those whose authority issues from a state less than fully conscious. Zen practice, for instance, places a high value on attaining simple spontaneity, "doing without thinking," which is the result of a breakthrough in consciousness, but this is a return to innocence rather than an operating from ignorance. The difference is enormous.

Another occasion for thanksgiving is reported in the story of the raising of Lazarus in the Gospel of John. This story is unique to this gospel and recounts the death of a personal friend of Jesus to whose home he had made many visits. The story is told in chapter 11 : 11–44, and involves great emotion including the famous verse, "Jesus wept." Just before raising Lazarus, Jesus says a prayer which begins, "Father, I thank thee. . . ." The phrase comes as a surprise to a reader of this story since, by usual standards, there seems little for which to be thankful. When

Lazarus' death is announced by Jesus his disciples do not understand what he is talking about. In going to bethany to be with Lazarus' sisters, Martha and Mary, Jesus is going back into country dangerous for him. Martha greets him with the words, "If you had been here, sir, my brother would not have died." When Mary finally arrives at the place where Jesus is she also accosts him with the words her sister used. Jesus breaks into tears and then is accused by the mourners who had gathered of not using his power to prevent the event from happening. He asks that the stone be rolled away from the tomb and is met with Martha's complaint that, since Lazarus had been dead for four days, there will be a stench caused by his decaying flesh. It is at this moment that Jesus offers thanks! For what? That he is "heard" by the Father, in communication, communion with the infinite. From that level of judgment he can see that "all things work together for good," (to quote Paul) that even in the midst of lack of understanding, complaints, the death of a loved one, personal grief, and public criticism there is occasion for thanksgiving. There is no moment in the divine economy unworthy of thanks because the order of the universe is bringing into balance that which seems extreme. Thanksgiving at times of difficulty is a powerful expression of trust in the basic goodness of creation. Jesus' trust is not without cause. Soon Lazarus stands at the entrance of the tomb, still wrapped in the cloths of burial: alive.

In Herman Aihara's booklet, *Seven Basic Macrobiotic Principles,* (not identical with the seven principles central to this work) he states:

> The fifth and most important principle of macrobiotics is *appreciation* (gratitude). Why? Because it is the cause of freedom and happiness. *Without it there can be no freedom or happiness.* (p. 13)

In a lecture at the 1984 Macrobiotic Summer Camp, held in the Berkshires of Massachusetts, Herman Aihara said that he had thought long and hard to come up with a physical condition which, in itself, promoted an attitude of gratitude. He decided that being hungry engendered thanks, rather than having a full and satisfied stomach. This fits well with the macrobiotic recommendation that one should eat only until two thirds full, and also squares with the universal religious practice of fasting. Being hungry, even just a little hungry, makes us think; gives us confidence in controlling our appetite at other times; reminds us of our dependency upon the creator of our food which, in turn, creates us, and since only those who have been hungry can know what hunger means, sensitizes compassion for those who are hungry. Being hungry promotes acknowledgement of our interconnectedness which is most appropriately expressed as thanksgiving. Thanksgiving is the antidote for arrogance.

The Interpreter's Dictionary of The Bible begins the section on gratitude with these words:

> No motif more adequately reveals the nature of biblical faith than does gratitude or thanksgiving.[11]

That strong statement of the centrality of expressed appreciation in the faiths of Judaism and Christianity, compared with the many references to the equivalent centrality of gratitude in other world religions and macrobiotics makes gratitude the universal meeting ground.

> Our gratitude will pave the way to Him, and shorten our learning time by more than you could ever dream of. Gratitude goes hand in hand with love, and where one is the other must be found. For gratitude is but an aspect of the Love which is the Source of all creation. God gives thanks to you, His Son, for being what you are; His Own completion and the source of love, along with Him. Your gratitude to Him is one with His to you. For love can walk no road except the way of gratitude, and thus we go who walk the way to God.[12]
>
> Be filled with the Spirit, addressing one another in psalms,

and hymns, and spiritual songs, singing and making melody to the Lord with all your heart, always and for everything giving thanks in the name of our Lord Jesus Christ to God the Father. (Ephesians 5: 18b–20)

---

[1] Aihara, *Seven Basic Macrobiotic Principles,* p. 14.
[2] quoted in Simcox, *A Treasury of Quotations on Christian Themes,* p. 3.
[3] Ohsawa, *Zen Macrobiotics,* p. 17.
[4] see Kushi, *The Book of Macrobiotics,* pp. 20 ff.
[5] for a full discussion see Chapter 7, Ohsawa, *The Book of Judgment,* p. 97.
[6] Michio Kushi Seminar Report, No. 8, pp. 16, 17.
[7] Starvation is only the symptom of the real disease—greed. Greed is a manifestation of arrogance, the belief in the illusion that each of us is separate. Arrogance is living a lie.
[8] It is apparent, however, in reading both Ohsawa and Kushi that the latter takes a considerably harder line in assigning these levels than the former. Such differences, like those contradictions which appear in sacred literature, only serve to call us to an awareness of the spirit of "I do not believe" or *non credo.* To be a true student of macrobiotics means to be responsible for generating one's own information through experience, taking what respected teachers offer on good report but using such information for guidance toward an "owned" knowledge.
[9] Wallace L. Chafe, *Seneca Thanksgiving Rituals,* Bureau of American Ethnology Bulletin 183, p. 1, notes that the word translated "greet," may also be translated, "thank, be thankful or grateful to or for, rejoice in, bless. . . ." It seems that "the Seneca concept is broader than that expressed by any simple English term, and covers not only the conventionalized amenities of both thanking and greeting, but a more general feeling of happiness over existence of something or someone."
[10] Tooker, *Native American Spirituality of The Eastern Woodlands,* p. 58.
[11] *Interpreter's Dictionary of The Bible,* Vol. 2, p. 470.
[12] *A Course in Miracles,* Vol. 2, p. 363.

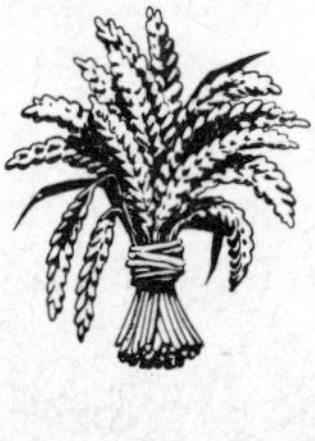

Chapter 10

Forgiveness

"Forgive and you will be forgiven."
(Luke 6: 37b)

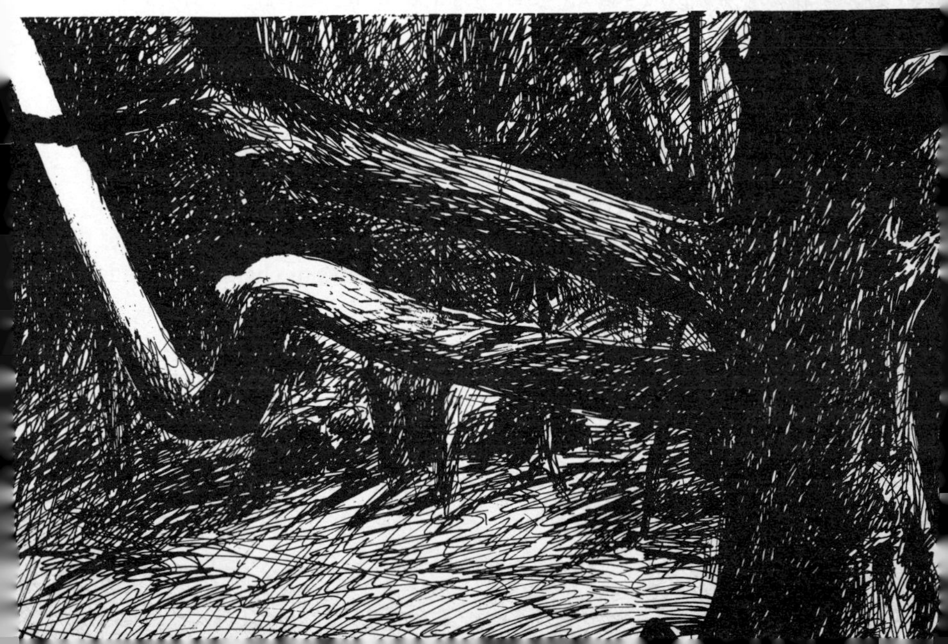

IN THE COURSE OF THIS BOOK the seven universal principles of macrobiotic philosophy have been discussed. The claim of their universality has been supported by their having been interpreted in the language and imagery of the Bible. Although these principles were enunciated and elaborated out of the philosophy of the orient, it is our claim that the truths to which they point may be described in the language of any culture. In applying these principles we have also discussed the universal concepts of polarity and gratitude, and in the next chapters will survey the necessary occurrence of awareness and self reflection—prayer, or meditation. However, this chapter deals with a uniquely biblical approach to a universal truth. The truth, found in the first principle of the infinite universe, is that of the unity of creation; an approach to its realization is forgiveness. Forgiveness heals the illusion of separation, or belief in the ultimate reality of the world of this and that. In the last chapter we saw the power of thanksgiving to effect the same result, the realization of unity, in the act of giving thanks. Thanksgiving is found at the heart of religious practice worldwide, but the centrality of forgiveness, elaborated so effectively in the life and teaching of Jesus, is unique to Christianity.

In Islam, the Koran describes a kind of forgiveness. In the post death experience falsehoods accumulated during earthly existence are described as being burned away as the self proceeds toward the beatific vision of unity. In Eastern thought the understanding of the impersonal nature of the cosmos precludes the very personal notion of one person, be that person divine or human, forgiving another. Forgiveness requires the possibility of choosing not to forgive, and in a universe playing out an infinite number of possibilities according to the laws of change, where is the possibility of choice? In addition to the mechanical interpretation of manifestation one confronts the difficulty of making a case for forgiveness in Eastern thought where ultimate reality is "nothing;" therefore, there is nothing to forgive. In the religion of India there is no image of forgiveness by a loving creator. Again, the idea is more mechanical: if you have done something wrong, you have to undo it. Balance is acheved by doing something good to undo the wrong. No one can forgive you. You are totally responsible for changing your karmas which accrue by your own actions. In macrobiotic philosophy place exists for this concept in spite of its Eastern origins. Self purification is seen as the way to the realization of unity. The delusion of separation is transcended by living according to the order of the universe. This position is described in a transcript of a 1975 Michio Kushi lecture:

> . . . when we sin we should review that we are doing and what we are thinking according to the order of the universe. With an empty mind we should come back to the center, and whatever we think we should say. Then heaven and earth will be very happy to hear that, and at the same time our delusions will disappear. This purification is taking care of sin. . . . and if we fail to enact our own purification no one will say anything. If we don't purify ourselves of our own sin, if we don't correct ourselves, then the order of the universe will naturally destroy us. We will become sick, or we will have an accident. There is no need to accuse anyone. There is no need to judge. That is the ancient idea of sin which comes to us from the Far East.[1]

One purpose of this book is the reconciliation of apparent divergences between macrobiotic philosophy and Christian theology. Why, then, is the concept of forgiveness included? Is this obvious divergence irreconcilable?

There could be no consideration of the spirit of Christianity without a discussion of forgiveness. Christianity is the inheritor of the religion which produced the words, "Bless the Lord, O my soul, and forget not all his benefits, who forgives all your iniquity, who heals all your diseases . . ." (Psalm 103:2, 3), and which looks to the teachings of the one who instructed his followers to pray, "Forgive us our sins as we forgive the sins of others." (Luke 11:4). Martin Luther said, "Forgiveness of sins is the heart of Christianity. . . ." The master, Jesus, at the end of his earthly life, when nails were being driven into his wrists said, "Father, forgive them, for they know not what they do," (Luke 23:34). Stephen, first Christian martyr, echoes Jesus' words as he is being stoned to death, "Lord, do not hold this sin against them," (Acts 7:60.)

The popular notion of forgiveness as practiced in the Christian religion is as far amiss as the idea that Christians believe that you should live a good life now so that you will go to heaven. The master Jesus would be appalled to think that his simple religion of the heart had been turned into a business deal complete with payoff! So, too, forgiveness as an act where the forgiver is considered superior to the forgiven as if to say, "I, the righteous one, forgive you, the sinner," is totally foreign to the biblical concept of forgiveness. Such a stance is pure arrogance and a veritable wallowing in the illusion of separation. This is an attitude which tells us more about the forgiver than about the offender and the offence.

The Old Testament use of forgiveness is concerned primarily with the "forgiveness" of humankind by the creator. In the anthropomorphic imagery of the Old Testament, humanity is seen as having separated itself from its origin by its own doing and blocked the return by barriers erected through disobedience. In macrobiotic rhetoric the condition is identically described as resulting from a failure to following the order of the universe. God then forgives or, in Hebrew, "sends away," "covers," "removes," "wipes away" those barriers, and thus restores union. The quality which effects this sending away is God's *chesed* or steadfast love: "Have mercy upon me, O God, according to thy steadfast love; according to thy abundant mercy blot out my transgressions," (Psalm 51:1). This same divine compassion is also translated "loving kindness," in other passages. The Septuagint, the Greek translation of the Old Testament, also uses the term "to send away." There is no superior God who stoops to sinful humankind, but there *is* a creator whose intrinsic nature is unity and whose creation, in truth, partakes of that nature, whose love is so vast "as to make even antagonisms complementary." The true nature of creation, at all levels, is seen as exhibiting qualities of the creator, (Romans 1: 19, 20); thus "sending away" is the order of the universe, the divine economy. To carry blatantly anthropomorphic imagery to its extreme, "God has a short memory." There is no anger or arrogance in covering up or sending away. As stones in the garden are tossed to the side, or infertile patches are covered with loam, those things which prevent the full flowering of the realization of unity are sent away and covered up. As Paul, so thoroughly trained in the Old Testament tradition, reminds his readers, "You are God's garden," (1 Corinthians 3: 9b). Each of us requires special cultivation in the form of sending away and covering up to bring our being to full flower.

The garden analogy breaks down rather quickly upon examination, however. The garden does not place its stones in the way or create infertile patches volitionally, nor does it require the conditions appropriate for intensive agriculture necessary for the garden of humanity to come to full fruition. But, just as the gardener goes about the tasks of making ready the soil so the created order, without malice or retribution, keeps our soil fertile for whatever seeds may be sown.

It is in the New Testament that forgiveness is woven so inextricably into the fabric of Christianity. The first mention of forgiveness in the gospels is in accordance with the Old Testament emphasis on divine activity. John Baptist comes "proclaiming a baptism in token to repentence for the forgiveness of sins," (Mark 1: 4). People can celebrate the "sending away" of those things which separate them from the creator by the ceremonial "washing away" in the water of baptism. It is also in the New Testament's view of forgiveness that we find the correlation to the "self-purification" of macrobiotic philosophy. Although the inspiration and power for the unifying act of forgiveness comes from the source of all inspiration, the Spirit within, there is still required a voluntary act on the part of the one who is forgiven to make the forgiveness complete. In fact, so necessary is the operation of the self, that forgiveness cannot occur without a conscious choice. In John The Baptist's preaching, the choice is for repentance or turning back from the path of error and choosing to enter the water to be baptized as a symbol of that act of repentance. There can be no forgiveness without the conscious choice having been made.

Jesus' teaching makes forgiveness totally dependent upon one's own doing:

> And when you stand praying, if you have a grievance against anyone, forgive him, so that your Father in heaven may forgive you the wrongs you have done. (Mark 11:25)

> Forgive us our sins as we forgive the sins of others. (Luke 11:4)

There is no forgiveness for the one who does not forgive; we are forgiven only as much as we forgive. It would be difficult to imagine how an activity could be more dependent upon the action of the self than those two descriptions of forgiveness. The purifying activity of forgiveness, then, is dependent upon each person's willingness to initiate the act, just as, in macrobiotic philosophy, self purification is undertaken by turning back and reviewing our difficulties in light of the order of the universe. In biblical understanding forgiveness is an integral part of the divine economy and is the process by which barriers to unity are "sent away." Forgiveness is, for Judaism and Christianity, an integral, inextricable part of the order of the universe.

Personal responsibility is stressed at every turn in the teachings of Jesus. "Your faith has cured you," follows most of the healings in which Jesus was involved. We are told to love our neighbors "as you love yourself." It is the publican, concerned only for righting his own shortcomings, who is justified in his prayer life, not the Pharisee who is thankful that he is not like the publican. Jesus asks why we are concerned with the speck of sawdust in our brother's eye while we have a plank in our own. The woman who anointed Jesus with precious oil while he was at dinner at a

Pharisee's home is forgiven her many sins because she has shown much love. Personal responsibility is also taught by the early preachers of the gospel: "Repent and be baptized, every one of you in the name of Jesus the Messiah for the forgiveness of your sins," Peter states, (Acts 2: 38). Again Peter says, "Repent then and turn to God, so that your sins may be wiped out," (Acts 3: 19). In Caesarea, Peter preaches, ". . . everyone who trusts in him receives forgiveness of sins through his name," (Acts 10: 43). Something must be done by the believer—repentance, baptism, trust. The voluntary turning back preached by John Baptist is a necessary part of the forgiveness process. This "turning back" meant by the word repentence can only be done by act of will in assurance that the power of grace to make the turn is there for anyone wishing to do so. Paul states that we are not tested beyond our ability to withstand, but that with the test a way out is provided by way of the strength to sustain the test, (1 Corinthians 10: 13). Such an assurance provides a foundation for confidence to follow Paul's injunction to "work out your own salvation . . ." (Philippians 2: 12).

In the act of turning back there is acceptance of personal responsibility for one's own condition. Ultimately, it is in the acknowledgment of responsibility that forgiveness is realized. The process cannot be divided into acceptance of responsiblity . . . repentence . . . forgiveness. Connectedness with what appears to be out there is established; unity is realized; forgiveness comes. In the very act of acknowledging responsibility and interdependence, then acting upon that acknowledgment, a whole process is set in motion which has the power to establish "the peace that passes understanding," (Philippians 4: 7) the peace of unity. This unitive experience is ineffable, beyond words, so much more than can be grasped by the intellect that Paul describes it as hearing "things that cannot be told, which man may not utter," (2 Corinthians 12: 4). For acknowledgment to be wholehearted there must be more than a tacit, intellectual recognition of responsibility but an acting upon that recognition by the whole person: "Be doers of the word and not hearers only, deceiving yourselves," (James

1:22). There is a self deception in intellectualizing which convinces the intellectualizer that his whole being is involved when, in reality, he is living only "from the neck up." A way of life is much more than a way of thinking, but it issues from one's thinking as well as informing one's ideas through the experiences of living.

Forgiveness, then, plays a prominent part in Jesus' teaching as well in his activity itself. His baptism by John was an act demonstrating inclusion in, and support for, the need for repentance and forgiveness. That ceremonial washing began Jesus' public ministry and his life wove many harmonies around the keynote of turning back from the perception of separation to the truth of being one with the Father. This truth, when experienced, brings the wholeness of health. In the healing of the paralytic who was carried to him, Jesus declared, "My son, your sins are forgiven," (Mark 2:5), in other words, those things which separate you from the Father within are sent away. At these words the man was healed, made whole. It is at this point of the story that the Old Testament use of forgiveness as something only given by God is reasserted by the experts on Hebrew scriptures, the lawyers. They accuse Jesus of blasphemy, saying, "Who but God alone can forgive sins?" Jesus then shows that there is such an intimate connection between the onset of disease and separation that saying, "Your sins are forgiven," is the same as saying, "Take up your bed and walk." Jesus then says to the paralytic, "Take up your bed and walk," and he does. Forgiveness is given a new and far deeper meaning.

The power to forgive is not restricted to the creator or even to a special manifestation of the creator, as Christians believe Jesus to be. Jesus, himself, commissions his disciples with the words, "If you forgive any man's sins they stand forgiven," (John 20:23). In answering Peter's question about how many times to forgive, it is understood not only that we are to forgive but that this forgiveness should be without limit (Matthew 18:21, 22). Forgiveness is shown to have the quality of unconditional giving when Jesus says, "Seventy times seven" as the number of times to forgive. He is definitely not saying that forgiveness should stop when one reaches four hundred ninety acts of forgiveness, but rather, that there must be no limit. There is no limit to the infinity of unity. The moment a limit to forgiveness is set and reached the illusion of separation begins again. We fall back into dualistic thinking, ego versus ego, and the misperception that we have been harmed by someone else rather than that any harm done is by ourselves to ourselves through our very misperception.

Forgiveness is central to what has come to be called the doctrine of the atonement, a universal in the preaching and teaching of the early church. The doctrine of the atonement asserts that Jesus' death was a sacrifice for the separation (sins) of the whole world, and by that act at-onement stands as an ever-present reality for all humankind. This is an easy doctrine to quote since it appears throughout the writings of Paul and has been written back into the teachings of Jesus by the believers who produced the gospels. However, the atonement is a particularly difficult doctrine to explain without appearing to place the total responsibility for our relationship with the universe on Jesus' shoulders, thus negating his obvious belief that it is by our voluntary response that conditions are established for unity to be realized. Even here, though, it is the act of faith on the part of the Christian which effects the new life of reconciliation between divinity and humanity. Nowhere in theology is the separateness of the divine and the human stressed more than in the doctrine of the atonement, the need for a sacrificial death, a propitiation for the sins of the whole world.

This doctrine issues from the fall/redemption theological tradition which has assumed a dominant position in Christian theology. However, there is a parallel tradition, of equally ancient origin, known as "creation spirituality." This celebration of the basic goodness of creation is found in all major religions and, someday, will form the basis of a global theology. This universal theme of creator revealed in creation is biblical and an underlying assumption of this volume on universals.[2]

The notion of the need for atonement was nourished by roots

which have their origin very deep in human history. Sacrificial death has been practiced by various cultures worldwide. The use of substitutes is mentioned in Babylonian magical ceremonies and Hittite rituals: Parts of the Book of Genesis which date to the fifth Century B.C. expound on the need for a "guilt offering." The famous story of Abraham and his son Isaac in Genesis 22, is a story of a sacrificial death. Abraham is called upon, as a test, to kill his son, "as a sacrifice" (22:2). Just as he is about to kill Isaac, he spies a ram caught by its horns in a thicket. He sacrifices the ram instead and his son is spared. Even in modern Arabic custom there is widespread use of the *fedu* or animal ransom. This ancient and primitive custom was in use at the time of Jesus in the form of the scapegoat upon which the sins of the people were ceremonially and symbolically heaped on the Day of Atonement before it was led off into the wilderness. At first this goat was simply led off to "a solitary land" (Leviticus 16:22). Later the ritual became more elaborate with reporting stations posted along the way to a precipice far from the village. When the goat was pushed over the cliff to its death, news was relayed back to the waiting throngs now purged of the miasma of their wrong doings. The scapegoat did not remove the responsibility of the sinner but bore on its back the negative energy, the taint of separation. The event took place at the opening of the agricultural year and was seen as a "spring cleaning" to make the whole community ready for the new life which lay before them.

The Babylonian festival of Akitu was celebrated at the beginning of a new year; on its fifth day a sheep was beheaded and the freshly cleaned and fumigated temple walls were rubbed with its carcass. This ceremony was called *kippuru* and is reflected in the Hebrew *Kippurim* meaning "purgation" or "atonement." The need for a ceremonial substitute and/or death lies deep in the traditions of the biblical countries. This need issued from the belief that there were barriers, conditions, subtle circumstances which needed to be wiped away in order for the road to be cleared to and from divine power.

The suffering servant passages in Isaiah stand as the most

obvious Old Testament precurser to the belief that "Christ died for the ungodly," and ". . . we have now been justified by Christ's sacrificial death . . ." (Romans 5:6, 9). The mysterious passage in Isaiah bursts upon the biblical scene without any obvious precedent and details the suffering of a servant of the Lord who:

> has borne our griefs and carried our sorrows . . . he was wounded for our transgressions, he was bruised for our iniquities . . . and with his stripes we are healed. (Isaiah 53:4, 5)

That a human being could suffer "as a ransom for all" (1 Timothy 2:6), was an idea ready for appropriation by the early Christian community. To see in the suffering and death of their master the fulfillment of Isaiah's prophecy was a natural interpretation of the crucifixion.

There could have been no resurrection without the crucifixion, so crucifixes depicting this agonizing and bloody form of capital punishment are used in Christendom as reminders of old life/new life, death/resurrection, cross/crown. This symbol has been seen by some as offensively grotesque. George and Lima Ohsawa were horrified by the crucifixes they encountered in France.[3] Mr. Ohsawa even ascribed the origin of cruelty in the West to the presence of these symbols. Michio Kushi relates a similar revulsion by Herman Aihara who couldn't sleep in the chapel of a friend because of the presence of a crucifix in the room.' Such incidents demonstrate well the backs and fronts principles. For the Christian believer, the back side of crucifixion is resurrection. To depict one is to depict the other. The crucifixion is seen as a symbol of great triumph, an acceptance of the truth of fronts and backs in accord with macrobiotic principles. However, for the stranger to such belief all that is seen is a bloody cadaver. In fact, the failure of Protestantism to grasp the universality of fronts and backs has resulted in the use of only the cross, without the corpus attached, in Protestant churches. Yet, the hallmark of fundamentalist Protestantism is the call to believe in the saving blood of Jesus for the forgiveness of sins. Many who preach such doctrine may well have no idea of the primitive nature of such a belief or of the use of similar theology in "pagan" religion.

The word "atonement" originates from the combination of two words: at-onement. The condition necessary for the realization of unity is purity of heart, mind, and body, the "sending away" of those things which stand in the way. Regardless of whether that "sending away" is conceptualized within an esoteric doctrine or is solely an act of self purification through dietary and spiritual practice, there must be a discharge of impediments to wholeness. Forgiveness offers a way to remember that all things proceed from one infinity, that in an everchanging universe, today's curse is changing into tomorrow's blessing, and that the perception of separation is a necessary and complementary other side of the realization of unity. The "sending away" which takes place in forgiveness marks the end of separation. Thus, all seven universal principles of the infinite universe are subsumed in the act of forgiveness. Because of complementarity, the act of forgiveness is also informed and enhanced by an understanding of the principles. Forgiveness naturally ensues when the principles come alive for us by being lived out from the heart. Awareness of unity is, itself, tantamount to forgiveness and is a remembering of our true nature as being at one with all of creation.

The central act of Christian worship must be included in this discussion as well. The ceremonial table fellowship established by Jesus and practiced throughout the history of the Church was recorded by the writer of Matthew as having been instituted with the words, "This is my blood of the new covenant, which is poured out for many for the forgiveness of sins," (Matthew 26:28). In the holy thanksgiving of eucharistic fellowship there is a "sending away," an establishment of the conditions for making whole. This holiness comes through an act of eating together, albeit ceremonially. In the thankfulness of the moment, forgiveness naturally ensures. The symptom of the perception of separation, arrogance, is "sent away" by the obvious inclusiveness and unifying power of food shared around a common table. Not only are the participants at a meal sitting together, but the quality of their internal physiological processes are aligned by partaking the same food. The truth of their unity is there to be grasped by all who will forgive: let go of the illusion of separation.

Forgetting is usually an involuntary act, but forgiveness is remembering to forget. A recent cartoon showed a very elderly man standing at the church door and saying to the minister, " 'Love your enemies', is a wonderful concept. The problem is that I can't remember who they are!" That man had already forgiven them by virtue of his forgetting. When the Moravian missionaries first went to the Eskimos they discovered that there was no word for forgiveness in the native tongue. They had to compound one and came up with an enormous assemblage of letters which hit upon the heart of the matter: issumagijoujungnainermik. It means: "not-being-able-to-think-about-it-anymore."

Forgiveness is letting go. Dr. Gerald Jampolsky, in his best seller, *Love is Letting Go of Fear*, gives an exercise in creative visualization or "active imagination," as he calls it, which is helpful in the "sending away" process. This exercise is designed to help us forgive ourselves by watching the emotional junk we have collected float away in a garbage pail suspended beneath a yellow, helium-filled balloon.[5] He suggests that, following the exercise, we be aware of how much lighter we feel. "Give, give, and give infinitely," says George Ohsawa. By so doing we become lighter and facilitate the ascent up the expanding spiral of judgment. Letting go is also a characteristic of life in the Kingdom of God. When we cling to the perception of past hurts forgiveness becomes impossible. We are putting our hand to the plow and looking back. We become as stuck as Lot's wife. There is a popular expression in some Christian circles which recognizes the power in faith or trust in the ability of the natural order of things to bring into balance what is lopsided: "Let go, and let God." As with a listing ship, ballast must be thrown overboard to keep us on an even keel. Forgiveness is throwing that ballast overboard.

Forgiveness brings us into the present without old emotional baggage. Any act which so engenders a sense of separation in us that it requires forgiving has already happened, is already in the past. The event cannot be changed, but it is possible to work with the effects upon us—anger, alienation, hurt, thoughts of retribution.

We can ask some questions which may help to put the act in perspective: did the offending party intend to offend? The answer to that one is often likely to be, "probably not." If we knew what led up to the commission of the offense—upbringing, state of health, the events immediately preceding the offense, etc., we might understand why such behavior occurred. Besides, perhaps the very act is being offered by a loving universe as an important lesson for us.

A question is sometimes heard as the offence scenario is reviewed, "Who does he think he is, anyway?" That really *is* the question—almost. Rather than the Pharisaical approach of being concerned for the other person, ("Thank God I am not like others"), we might try the question on ourselves: "Who do I think I am?" or "Who am I?" If pursued relentlessly, this question must bring each of us to the realization that all of the former questions were sheer silliness, pure egoistic sentimentality, products of a gross failure to recognize what even a child knows innately before being introduced to the perception of separation—that ultimately there is no one to offend and no one to forgive. The vital energy which produces what I perceive to be offensive in you is the same energy which is forgiveness in me. Sometimes it is offence, sometimes it is forgiveness. If it is offence that we see then we must engage in some form of "sending away" to participate consciously in the balance toward which all things move.

Answers can help to put questions to rest and to give us breathing room to just let things be, but they can also pave a path to go "astray into a wilderness of words," (1 Timothy 1:6). When personal events are called into question, the question "why did this happen to me?" is seldom appropriate. The question, "What do I do now?" is invariably appropos. When mechanical failures occur, the question "why?" is always appropriate, but there is more to the tremendously complex constellation of factors in personal action and reaction than those in the pure model of Newtonian mechanics. If the personal event is a joyful one, the answer to "What do I do now?" is: rejoice. If the event is a negative one, resist the urge to obsess in the subjunctive tense; forgive yourself and others who participated in it, and recognize it as a lesson in the results of imbalances. Then, responding to the challenge of the lesson's questions, investigate the details of the lesson, arrive at answers which can be acted upon without using categories of "good" and "bad." The issue is not how to protect the ego but what enables a movement toward balance.

Salvation and forgiveness are inseparable. The perception of good and evil is the illusion from which we are to be saved. It was the arising of this perception, depicted biblically in the story of Adam and Eve's eating of the fruit of the tree of the knowledge of good and evil, which caused the illusion of separation. This illusion is dispelled by the unifying circle of forgiveness.

I recently heard a "from the mouths of babes" story which illustrates the point far more succinctly than abstract postulations. Leaving on vacation early one Sunday morning, a father asked the family whether or not they thought God would mind if they missed Church that day. The five year old immediately answered, "God doesn't mind anything!" To that can only be added, "Be ye perfect even as your father in heaven is perfect."

---

[1] Michio Kushi Seminar Report, No. 7, p. 28.
[2] For a full and excellent discussion of these two, parallel traditions see *Original Blessing, A Primer in Creation Spirituality,* by Matthew Fox.
[3] See George Ohsawa's *Jack and Mitie in the West* Chapter 2, The Origin of Cruelty in the West.
[4] Michio Kushi Seminar Report, No. 7, p. 29.
[5] Jampolsky, *Love is Letting Go of Fear,* p. 113.

Chapter 11

Awareness

"Awake, O sleeper. . . ." (Ephesians 5: 14)

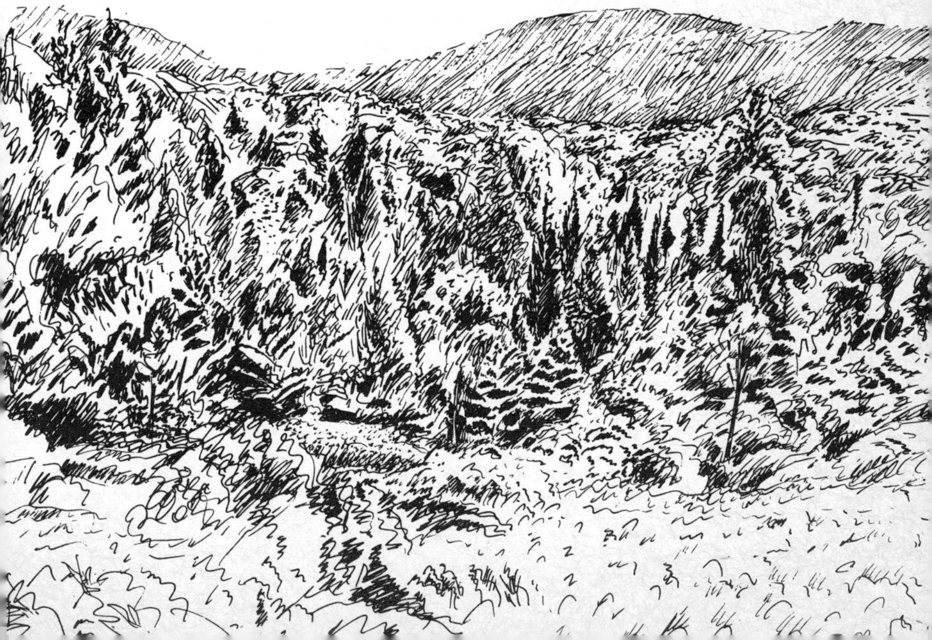

WOODY ALLEN HAS SAID, "Ninety percent of life is showing up." If you are not there you cannot get in the action. As obvious as that may sound, all of us miss a good deal of what is going on because we are somewhere else even when our bodies are where we want them to be. We may be doing the necessary four hours of daily day dreaming, rehearsing what we are going to say when it is our turn, thinking about the relaxing evening ahead, or thinking about the evening before, but we are "off on a cloud." One of the songs which came out of the drug culture of the sixties is Shel Silverstein's, *Got Stoned and Missed It*. The title is self explanatory, but the fact is that we can also be drugged by ego needs, by a desire to hold onto and live in the past, by looking forward to the promise of the future and in so doing miss the present. The issue is not "got stoned," but *missed it*.

The fact that we can be someplace in the body and not in spirit, or consciousness, is both a blessing and a curse. As far as we know this condition is peculiar to human beings and is part of what makes us human. Therefore, the common experience of estrangement from the present is one of the opportunities for greater growth offered by this dynamic creation for our benefit. The blessing is in the lesson and in the use of "elsewhereness" at times when the present appears unbearable to us because we have forgotten that all antagonisms proceed in a complementary and everchanging way from one infinity. Using "elsewhereness" to escape the moment by intentional daydreaming is a blessing only in so far as we can become aware of it and return to the moment. The curse of temporal estrangement is that it is possible to live our whole lives, never being fully where we are, and miss a whole lifetime. This also means that when we come to that last event in life—our death—we will miss that, too, and to miss our death means not knowing where we are in the life to come. No wonder *awareness* is an esteemed, transcultural value held in the highest regard by all the great religions of the world.

The word translated "sin" in both the Hebrew and the Greek simply means "to miss." Eliphaz tells Job not to despise what

God is doing to him because there will be rewards in his realization of unity with the created order (Job 5:23) and further states that Job will "inspect your sheepfold and miss nothing," (Job 5:24). The word "miss" here is that used for "sin" elsewhere. The "sin" of separation from the infinite is committed when we "miss." Repentence is awareness of the "miss" and an active willingness to try not to miss. Temporal "missing" means separation because Truth can only be found in the moment and living in the past or the future means removal from the Truth. To repent or turn back is to become aware, to come to one's senses, to to recognize that an existential divergence has occurred and to take responsibility for the realignment.

The classic story of abandoning delusion and returning to realization of the truth is that of the Prodigal Son, (Luke 15: 11–32). Verse 16 describes the moment of realization that the life this young man was pursuing was unedifying, to say the least, with the words, "When he came to himself. . . ." Other translations use, "When he came to his senses. . . ." All agree that this act was one of a gathering of awareness to one point, whether described as sensory or ontological. To "come to one's self" means to be wholly in one place, a gathering of all qualitative and quantitative faculties. It is a state of being in the now. In the case of the prodigal son, he abandoned his delusion of future fulfillment as he reflected on the results of behavior motivated solely by expectation. This all began for him because he was sick of life on the farm and thought that life would be more exciting far away in a "distant country," that the future in some other place looked better than the present on the farm. At the moment that "he came to himself" he was "starving to death" (Luke 15:17) and eating the food he was feeding to the pigs he had been hired to oversee. Realization of his situation resulted in a turning back, a repentence, and return to his father and the farm. Once pride, arrogance, and other ego needs are set aside, the return becomes easy. The Father always welcomes the one who has come "to himself" in the same way that the father of the prodigal welcomed him: "While he was still a long way off his father saw him, and his heart went out to him. He ran to meet him, flung his arms round him, and kissed him," (Luke 15:20). The difficult part is "coming to." Once that is done the now is not just waiting with an open arms welcome but running to meet us while we are "still a long way off."

Awareness and repentence are different aspects of the same action. There is a turning back in awareness by the very fact that one has "come to." In both awareness and repentence there is a waking up from the dream world of past and future to a realization of the power of the ever changing, ever revitalized now. For the inflexible personality there may be some consolation in clinging to the petrified succession of nows (thens) represented by the past. They give the illusion of a static world of phenomena. The same consolation may be provided by building a thought form of the future replete with details which include prerequisites for its attainment. The same inflexible personality who is "bent out of shape" by a disagreeable interpretation of the past feels duty-bound to force the present to unfold as required by the dictates of the thought form of the future. Simply to be aware that attachment to either past or future exists is the beginning of the repentance process, a beginning of the return to the now. One of the surprising results of awareness is breaking the power of habitual thought patterns by the very act of identifying those patterns as arising. They fall away as a dream recedes in intensity when we move in consciousness from the world of sleep to the world of wakefulness.

Sensory perceptions cease when we are asleep. We are no longer in our bodies whose senses perceive this world. We are even said to be, "dead to the world." Sleep is a New Testament euphemism for death; we seem to be dead while asleep. When Lazarus died, Jesus said, "Our friend Lazarus has fallen asleep," (John 11:11). His disciples took him literally. Paul describes the second coming in 1 Corinthians as manifesting to both those who are alive and those who are dead, with the words, "we shall not all sleep," (1 Corinthians 15:51). Earlier in the chapter he speaks of those who have died as, "those who have fallen asleep,"

(1 Corinthians 15:20). To be asleep, dreaming in the past or the future, is to be dead to the now. So the writer of Ephesians rouses his readers with the words, "Awake, O sleeper, and arise from the dead, and Christ will give you light," (Ephesians 5:14). This quote comes from a passage admonishing believers who are very much alive. This is not directed to the physically dead but the existentially estranged, who, blinded by the darkness of sleep, cannot see that they are "children of light," (Ephesians 5:8). This theme echoes 1 Thessalonians, where Paul equates being "sons of light" with being in the daylight. Therefore, his readers are not to exhibit nighttime behavior, sleep and drunkenness. "Let us not sleep, as others do, but let us keep awake and be sober," (1 Thessalonians 5 : 6). Paul's similar admonition in Romans 13:11, 12, is one of the more famous quotes from that book:

> Besides this you know what hour it is, how it is full time now for you to wake from sleep. For salvation is nearer to us now than when we first believed; the night is far gone, the day is at hand. Let us then cast off the works of darkness and put on the armor of light.

Death and sleep, repentence and wakefulness are equated in The Book of Revelation:

> I know your works; you have the name of being alive, and you are dead. Awake, and strengthen what remains and is on the point of death. . . . Remember, then, what you have received and heard; keep that and repent. If you will not awake, I will come like a thief, and you will not know at what hour I will come upon you. (3:1b–3)

Again, in Chapter 16, verse 15, we find:

> Lo, I am coming like a thief! Blessed is he who is awake. . . .

How often has each of us been the recipient of the not too gentle admonition, "Wake up!" This reminder to "be here now," is a call to awareness which echoes through the New Testament. In the calls to repentence by John Baptist, in Jesus' announcing of the dawn of the kingdom, in the preaching of the apostles and the early Church fathers, "Wake up!" is the theme.

Katha Upanishad 3, 14 admonishes "Arise, wake up! Be vigilant, since you have received the 'gifts!' " The precise meaning of the name Buddha is "The Awakened One."

One of the most obvious differences between being awake and being asleep is the power to see the world of wakefulness. In biblical times, watchmen were appointed to keep their watches over fields and vineyards through the night at harvest time. While others slept, the watchmen kept awake. City walls also had watchmen posted whose presence was especially necessary at times of siege, (Jeremiah 51:12). It is no wonder, then, that the Bible uses the figure of the watchman as appropriate to those who are mindful, aware, attentive. A watchman is awake while others sleep; a watchman sees danger and gives warning before it is too late. Just by being there a watchman discourages dangerous and disruptive behavior; a watchman waits and watches, patiently observes; a watchman sees:

> I wait for the Lord, my soul waits, and in his word I hope; my soul waits for the Lord more than watchmen for the morning, more than watchmen for the morning. (Psalm 130:5, 6)

The prophets who stand before God for the people and before the people for God, are likened to watchmen:

> Son of man, I have made you a watchman for the house of Israel; whenever you hear a word from my mouth, you shall give them warning from me. (Ezekiel 3:17)

Isaiah describes false prophets with these enlightening words:

> His watchmen are blind, they are all without knowledge; they are all dumb dogs, they cannot bark; dreaming, lying down, loving to slumber. (Isaiah 56: 10)

Jesus uses the metaphor of one who watches in his many calls to constant vigilance and awareness, admonishing his hearers to watch, to be awake and aware:

> Watch therefore—for you do not know when the master of the house will come, in the evening, or at midnight, or at cockcrow, or in the morning—lest he come suddenly and find you asleep. And what I say to you I say to all: Watch. (Mark 13: 35)

When the master of a house returned from a journey there was great rejoicing and feasting. Those who were asleep missed out on the fun.

The parables of the man who sowed good seed and then slept while an enemy came and sowed weeds, (Matthew 13: 25) and of the ten virgins, five of whom were not ready when the wedding party began are calls to awareness. Luke combines the marriage story and the story of the return of the master with the following words:

> Let your loins be girded and your lamps burning, and be like men waiting for their master to come home from the marriage feast, so that they may open to him at once when he comes and knocks. Blessed are those servants whom the master finds awake when he comes; truly, I say to you, he will gird himself and have them sit at table, and he will come and serve them. . . . You also must be ready; for the son of man is coming at an hour you do not expect. (Luke 12: 36–40)

These words refer to the end time and the need to be ready, since it may come "as a thief in the night." However, we have seen that the teaching of Jesus and the early Church was one of realized eschatology and, therefore, the call to watchfulness is a call to awareness in the here and now.

The quality of the awareness of a watchman is that of being wide awake, listening and watching with every fiber of being for the thief, the attackers, or the master of the house—as if one's life depends upon it. Indeed, one's life does depend upon this mode of consciousness, or, be it perceived as positive or negative, what happens in the now may be missed. Life may be missed!

In the collection of quotations from the masters of spiritual growth known as the desert fathers, fourth century Christian monks in the Egyptian desert, we find the following:

> Abba Bessarion, at the point of death, said, "The monk ought to be as the Cherubim and Seraphim: all eye."[1]

A number of expressions which allude to reality involve visual terminology. When we understand, we say, "I see." When we do not understand someone's behavior we say, "I can't see why he would do a thing like that." Many a child's demands have been put off with the words, "We'll see," meaning that the actuality, when it arrives, will be seen. In disagreements someone may say, "see here, now!" which is just another way of saying, "see things my way." Optical illusions aside, the eye can be trusted; "seeing is believing." Meister Eckhart reminds us of the unity of creation demonstrated in the act of seeing by saying, "The eye with which I see God is the very eye with which God sees me." The confirmation of the resurrection of Jesus was in seeing him, (Matthew 28:17, Luke 24:39, John 20:20). Thomas would not believe that the other disciples had seen the risen Jesus unless he saw the nail prints in Jesus' hands himself, (John 20:25).

The call to awareness is a call to active participation in perception, a literal and figurative call to see. The question is: what are we on the lookout for? The answer is: everything. We are to be watchmen watching.

We are to watch for the tendency to be lured out of the present by memories of the past and by either fond hopes or nagging doubts about the future. Each of us has an enormous library of material in our memory documenting all of our experiences, learnings, and daydreams. At any moment our brain, described by some as a bio-computer, is more than willing to feed its voracious appetite for constant activity by retrieving related material which it will play for us like tapes. It will splice and edit, cut and paste, revamp and replay. These tapes are not only of the past; we also have created tapes of the future, some of which we identify with so much that when the future becomes the present and disagrees with the prerecorded tape we suffer deep disappointment. The difficulty arises not because we had the expectation or made the plan or dreamed the dream but that we became so attached to it. For this reason many religions teach the importance of non-attachment. This teaching is found in Christianity in many sayings, one of which is, "The love of money is the root of all evil," (1 Timothy 6: 10). The problem is "the love of money," not the money.

The more often we allow certain tapes to play, the more accessible they become, and the more they occupy our thinking time. Without exercising awareness and volitionally intervening we can become obsessed with our attachments. An obsession is a playing of the same thought form over and over. The pattern must be broken for our own health's sake. This can be done by consciously diverting the thoughts which follow that pattern by becoming aware of their arising before we identify with them and they become all consuming.

Frequently the tendency to obsess is a danger during the process of grief. When we lose anything in life we grieve, whether it is a small loss or the significant loss through death of someone we love. A recognized stage in the grief process is the tendency to become obsessed with images of that which is lost. For example, we may use some particular scenario to remember a person who has died. As this scenario is repeated it becomes the only and constant memory. This is tantamount to getting stuck and is a phenomenon of which all grief counselors become aware.

Being stuck in mental processes can produce as much panic as being stuck on a railroad crossing. When the obsessive memories arise they should be acknowledged the way we acknowledge people who enters a room while we are reading. We let them go their way without engaging them in the diversion of conversation.

We are to observe attitudes and feelings as they arise in us and acknowledge their arising without being "carrried away" by those which only lead us to what should have been rather than what is. Gratitude is an attitude which fittingly celebrates the moment as the conscious receiving of the blessing of the now. Forgiveness restores us to the now by releasing us from the past. Love encompasses all moments as active participation in the now by being, in Brother David Steindl-Rast's words, "a wholehearted 'yes' to belonging."[2] Anxiety and its objectification, fear, are future oriented. They give our minds something to work on; but doing more than recognizing their arising leads us from the reality of the now to the "what if's" of the future. The First Epistle of John puts fear and love in their appropriate places by saying,

> There is no fear in love, but perfect love casts out fear. For fear has to do with punishment, and he who fears is not perfected in love. (1 John 4: 18)

This is the same epistle which identifies God with love, ". . . God is love" (1 John 4: 8b). In associating fear with future punishment John, in his First Epistle, also recognizes that things befall us for reasons other than personal, anthropomorphic vindictiveness on the part of the creator. We are not punished, but we may be reminded. If the gentle reminder has not caught our attention, then a less delicate one may be used. Rather than the gentle reminder of fatigue we may have to be moved on to the more compelling experience of chronic or even acute symptoms of pain or disease.

Without an awareness informed by the seven principles, pain and disease are seen as difficulties about which we complain rather than ones for which we give thanks. The usual report of the diagnosis is, "I'm afraid that I have heart disease," instead of an offering of thanks that there has been a reminder to reduce the intake of fats and oils and adopt a more relaxed and natural life style.

In this instance the principles apply in the following ways. First: disease arises from the source of all that is. It is not a capricious attack from the outside. The first principle reminds us that there is no "outside," that everything proceeds from one infinity. Disease is not the result of bad luck but of insufficient understanding of the universe. Second: lack of awareness of universal change is the cause of pessimistic resignation and, ultimately, of giving up the will to live. Body cells heal themselves when bathed in the vitality of qualitatively and quantitatively balanced blood. That there must be a destructive "disease process" with a "negative patient outcome" are modern medicine's euphemisms for "we don't understand what's going on." The second principle advises us that what is broken may become whole, or, on the other hand, early symptoms may change into disease. It is our choice to follow the way of life or the way of death. Third: the principle of complementarity reminds us that imbalances manifesting as disease have arisen as a natural result of the body trying to correct other imbalances. We are not being "attacked." We, ourselves, have generated the condition. Fourth: the principle of nonidenticalness points to the uniqueness of the particular disease arisen out of our unique condition. The particular course of treatment—diet, external applications, lifestyle changes, spiritual practices—must be unique as well. There are no easy answers spelled out for us to follow. We must bring tremendous awareness to bear on our own situation in order to ascertain what is appropriate in changing our particular manifestation of disease. Fifth: the fifth and sixth principles of backs and fronts offer great hope for the person who finally comes to awareness in the throes of deep disease. The unavoidable back side of the diseased front is a complementary state of health. Sixth: the seventh principle tells us that, between the beginning and end of the life of the body, there will be the beginning and end of trillions of changes. Some of these changes will be the arising of reminders of imbalances, or symptoms. These symptoms, if unattended to, may develop into full-blown disease. Disease is only a complex of related symptoms, of indicators or reminders, and it also ends when the underlying imbalance producing them ends. To suppress disease by treating symptoms does not address the real issue: What is the nature of the imbalance?

We are aware of those parts of our bodies which have the greatest concentrations of nerve endings, the lips and fingertips for instance. But the body functions as a whole, and symptoms of imbalance may present themselves only to be overlooked because of our inability to hear the warning. Moshe Feldenkrais titles a chapter in his book, *Awareness Through Movement*, "Becoming Aware of Parts of which We are not Conscious with the Help of Those of which We are Conscious."[3] Exercises are presented in the chapter which assist in bodily awareness and, therefore, help wake us from the anesthesia produced by years of ignoring the gentle reminders.

In their book, *Natural Birth Control, A Guide to Contraception through Fertility Awareness*, Katia and Jonathan Drake outline the complex but orderly process by which human ova are produced and, in the absence of fertilization, are discharged. They suggest keeping track of the basal temperature through the monthly cycle, checking cervical mucus and position,[4] and developing an awareness of the peculiarities of each woman's cycle. This excellent book is must reading for every woman of childbearing age and its methods offer a program for generating awareness of bodily processes which extend far beyond the reproductive cycle. By practicing bodily awareness the profound effect of environmental factors on the body becomes apparent. The indicators are affected by travel, climate, diet, emotional stress, physical activity, the time of the month, and even the time of day. Proof, indeed, that beings and their environment are not two!

The postures of Hatha Yoga offer a gentle stretching effect which facilitates awareness of the obvious changes in flexibility from session to session. The body is in a much different state later in the day than in the early morning. Sometimes "knots" get tied in usually flexible muscles or one side of the body will be more relaxed than the other. A regular regimen of Hatha postures will point out both subtle and obvious changes in the body. When compared with dietary patterns the effect of food on flexibility is readily recognizable.

Awareness is an inclusive rather than exclusive consciousness. It is expansive rather than contractive. Although awareness may be concentrated, in its fullest sense it is open to everything. It is said that when Zen meditation is properly entered into, the meditator can perceive the opening of a door a half inch into the room. This is very different from the exclusive form of meditation which encourages the meditator to leave the bodily senses behind and move to higher realms. Full awareness is a macroscopic phenomenon. It is the big view of the big picture rather than the little or tunnelled view of only a detail.

Inclusive awareness precludes feelings of sentimentality, for instance, by revealing the whole. For sentimentality to exist there must be an exclusive consciousness which, in James Breech's words, "selects only certain aspects of experience to the exclusion of all others in order that it might retain uncomplicated feelings about the phenomenon."[5] Such a definition explains why the sentimental level of judgment is only the third of seven levels in macrobiotic philosophy. Sentimentality is a function of the tender emotions like pity or nostalgia. Pity permits us to cling to the illusion of separation. Nostalgia encourages us to cling to the past by retrieving past emotions. Both exclude the now until pity eolves into compassion and nostalgia becomes grateful remembrance. Sentimentality is an adult's regression into the mental world of the child. Experiments by Piaget and others have proven that the ability to abstract grows as we grow until we reach the age upon which the Stanford-Binet Intelligence Quotient of 100 is based—fifteen years old. In one experiment with six year olds, Paiget had his subjects watch as he poured identical glasses of milk into two differently shaped containers. Every child said the container in which the milk rose highest had the most milk even though the milk in both containers was seen being poured from similar glasses identically full. Such reasoning is exclusive of even the most rudimentary logic, not because of a pathological lack of awareness but because of the lack of abstractive ability appropriate to the development levels of that age group. It is a simplistic consciousness which only sees the final result. After normal growth the child is able to see that there is more to the experiment than meets the eye. Further maturation brings with it the ability to comprehend the complexity of the situation—a more inclusive awareness. When an adult clings to the exclusive and childish consciousness of sentimentality, the fullness of life and joy in the enternal now is missed.

How can we develop awareness? How can we remind ourselves to be where we are, body and soul, to "show up" and not miss the moment? It is possible simply to put our minds to it and go ahead, to become aware that we have not been aware and to encircle the moment with previously drifting psychic energy. This is a self perpetuating process which becomes easier with practice. Perhaps we can use something as a reminder or guide. Prayer beads are used in many religions to assist in counting prayers and in keeping the mind of the worshipper on the subject. The little round stickers with two eyes and a smiling mouth are found stuck here and there many years after their initial popularity because they remind us to lighten up.

However, for the person really convinced of the power and necessity of awareness and of the appropriateness of "sin" as a translation for the Hebrew and Greek words "to miss," there is a whole discipline devoted to the subject of mindfulness: Vipassana meditation. The word "Vipassana" means to see things clearly. Vipassana comes out of the Buddhist tradition and evolved as a method of developing, according to Buddha's teaching, the first and most important of seven factors of enlightenment—mindfulness. In this meditation discipline there are four areas to which mindfulness may be applied: breath, feelings, consciousness and Dharma (the order of the universe or the law of God).

Macrobiotic practice is a form of meditation on the order of the universe, and one wonders if the psalmist was not involved in the same practice when the following was penned, ". . . his delight is in the law of the Lord, and on his law he meditates day and night," (Psalm 1:2). Consider also the advice of the Lord to Joshua just before he fought the battle of Jericho, "This book of the law shall not depart out of your mouth, but you shall meditate on it day and night . . ." (Joshua 1:8). George Ohsawa's definition of faith as knowledge of the unique principle, which he equated with divine justice, is a call to knowing by being aware of the orderly interplay of yin and yang.

If someone calls to you across a busy street at rush hour the greeting may not even be heard. If the same call comes during the afternoon lull some of the message may be understood. If the street is empty of traffic the call may be understood completely even if made in conversational tones. In Vipassana meditation the street is emptied of traffic by sitting in silence with attention directed only to the person calling us. The object of awareness usually suggested for beginning practice is an aspect of body function, and the most obvious is the breath. Breathing is always with us and it changes with our mental processes and levels of physical activity. When we sit quietly the breath can be observed either as it enters and exits the nose or as the abdomen rise and falls with each breath. This practice is not easy at first since the mind is always willing to come up with endless numbers of reasons why we could be doing something else or, since we are committed to sitting quietly, how many other things we could fasten our attention upon. As the process is watched, the attempts of the mind to throw up alluring thoughts worthy of attachment and pursuit becomes almost hilarious. However, to laugh at the attempt is to become attached to the nature of the offering and is a form of clinging, not letting go. The thoughts should simply be noted as, "Well, there's anxiety," or "Here comes fear." All the while the breath is followed. Since there is no such thing as Buddhist breath versus Christian breath, the Vipassana practice is universally applicable and a great tool. When thrown off balance by some event, being mindful of only the breath can offer powerful assistance in bringing one back toward center. The suggestion of counting to ten when upset is a similar technique. Both offer space in which to collect scattered energies.

If the rapid growth of fast food chains and TV dinners has said anything about American culture, it has been an eloquent comment on lack of awareness in food selection, preparation, and consumption. A tremendous opportunity for growth in awareness lies in conscious participation in each step of the process of feeding ourselves. This process determines the quality of our lives as we select the quality of the very stuff out of which we are made. Personal responsibility begins here. When we cannot feed ourselves by wide awake participation in the creation process we turn lives over to those who care less about us than we do about ourselves. It does not require superhuman insight to see that when we have planted seeds, tended and overseen nourishment of the plant, watched it grow, harvested it, and prepared it for cooking with grateful attention to its growth patterns, this food is of different quality from chemically fertilized, machine planted, cultivated, and harvested food, impersonally cooked in "short order" and served by a waitress who sees us as just another customer. This difference in quality also produces a difference in the quality of the person who eats it. A popular television program featuring films of people who were unwittingly photographed once featured a sequence taken in a fast food restaurant showing a man eating a hamburger who, literally, never chewed. He just took a bite and swallowed. He bolted his food like a dog. He never knew what he was eating. Beyond the issues of conscious production and preparation is the issue of how we eat our food.

Let us review the process of feeding ourselves with an eye to awareness of quality and attentiveness to the fact that in consuming food we are creating who we are—happy or sad, active or lethargic, calm or violent, whole or broken. In selecting foods we should look for those which are in the whole state rather than refined, as close to the way they came out of the ground as possible. Are they still alive? If we planted them would they grow?

If we can answer, "yes," to those questions all the better. This is why whole grains are preferred over fractured ones, and whole vegetables selected over those previously prepared and preserved. If the answer is, "no," then the question, "How is the food preserved?" must be asked. Drying is preferable to freezing, pickling in water and sea salt over canning, and certainly over the newly proposed process of irradiation. Color and texture should be appreciated as the food is prepared, and particular attention should be paid to the growth patterns inherent in the plant. These appear as lines such as those around pumpkin and squash. I once attended a two hour cooking class taught by Lima Ohsawa in which the first hour was devoted to analyzing the way the vegetables grew and how they should be cut during preparation. The work area should not be a busy street! The kitchen should be a place of calm and order, neat and clean, no chaotic background music on the radio, truly the room in which "the bread from heaven which gives life to the world" is transmuted into "daily bread," the meeting place of heaven and earth. The care with which the food is prepared will be communicated to those who consume it through the medium of the very food itself.

Just as the food should not be processed, the heat over which it is cooked should be unprocessed, too. Wood heat is best, but is generally unavailable to those in urban areas these days. This is just one more reason to move to the country! The evenness of wood stove heat is indescribable. Open flame is the next choice, and that includes gas. "Now you're cooking with gas!" was an expression which became popular as this country made the transition from wood stoves, meaning that one was modernizing. Had it stopped there perhaps we might all be better off. Electric heat is heavily processed energy. Coal, oil, or nuclear fission generated radiant energy is released into water to make steam for turning turbines to generate electricity which can then heat the coil on which the pan sets. Microwaves are electrical energy processed even further away from the flame. In fact, so processed is micro wave cooking that it really does not work on any food as unprocessed as whole grain. The more processed the food which is put into the microwave, the better appears the result. It seems terrific for frozen food.

What is the problem with processed food? In addition to being devitalized, it has the effect of producing processed people—out of touch with the earth, removed from their roots, afloat, preserved, but not fully alive. It becomes difficult to get one's feet on the ground to gain perspective in decision making; it is difficult to see the whole picture. Of processed vegetable quality foods are combined with food of animal origin, then we may well have a difficult time expressing our most basic human qualities—compassion, forgiveness, gratitude, language. "Why Johnny Can't Read" may not just be the teacher's fault.

If you do not believe that you are what you eat then much of the above will sound most absurd. However, please be sure that you have experiential evidence before condemning such a possibility out of hand. It will not take long to prove or disprove the basic theory, but it is an area of understanding which really deserves an attempt.

Now we come to the best part of the exercise—eating with awareness. Most of us have had practice for this in simply being a good guest, noticing the food which our host has offered and savoring it. However, full awareness requires more. It is the habit in Christian monasteries to take the meal in silence or while a lector reads from scripture or devotional literature. The food can be appreciated, each mouthful chewed thoroughly, and the meal invested with the energy which attention to gratitude brings. Notice the color of the food against the plate, the arrangement of the tableware and the delicate tracings which the energy patterns made as the food was growing. Recognize that this food is the distillation and concentration of the basic, subtle, creative energies out of which all the universe is constructed. These finer forces come to us in this beautiful and tasty form, and just as we savor our food and chew it thoroughly we will foster creation of a being who savors all of life, works through life's opportunities, bites off only what can be chewed. Anything which enhances the dining experience should be encouraged: positive topics of conversation, "atmosphere," unhurried courses. Gratitude should be expressed at the beginning and at the end of each meal to those who made the meal possible, especially to the Creator who produced such a joyful way to maintain life. Each meal taken with friends is a demonstration of the unity we share as we actually create one blood quality by sharing food of the same quality. Eating with awareness provides a solid foundation on which can grow a structure of awareness fit to house the universe.

As awareness of the moment comes more frequently the realization also comes that there is One deep within our being who sees and who savors, a watchman and witness, unattached and free. This One is the witness who has been there for as long as we can remember and, some would say, for as long as there has been a creation. This witness is the one whose identity we have known all of our lives. Think of your earliest memory. Who was it who perceived the world that day? You remember that one as you and yet there is hardly a cell left in your body or a thought in your mind which was there then. The whole universe is in a much different place; the planet earth is millions of miles from where it was then; nothing is the same. Relationships have come and gone; love and hate, joy and sorrow have shared your days and nights. Yet you remember the moment of so long ago and recognize that it was you who was there then and you who lived all of those intervening years and witnessed the everflowing change. Someone was there whom you knew and still know as you, unchanging, watching, ultimately unaffected by the swirling interplay of energy which has produced so much change. This One is the watchman with whom increased conscious contact brings increased insight, always seeing the now, moving through time seeing only the moment from the still point where the arms of the cross intersect. This witness sees the whirling wheel from the emptiness of the center of the hub and watches the temporal and the eternal with the same eye; "It is the Spirit himself, bearing witness with our spirit that we are children of God . . ." (Romans 8:16). This One is only met on the path of the way of life.

[1] Ward, *The Desert Christian,* p. 42.
[2] Steindl-Rast, *Gratefulness, The Heart of Prayer,* p. 206.
[3] Feldenkrais, *Awareness Through Movement,* p. 155.
[4] Drake and Drake, *Natural Birth Control,* Chapters 2, 3, & 4.
[5] Breech, *The Silence of Jesus,* p. 44.

Chapter 12

Self-Reflection

"Let us test and examine our ways,
and return to the Lord!" (Lamentations 3:40)

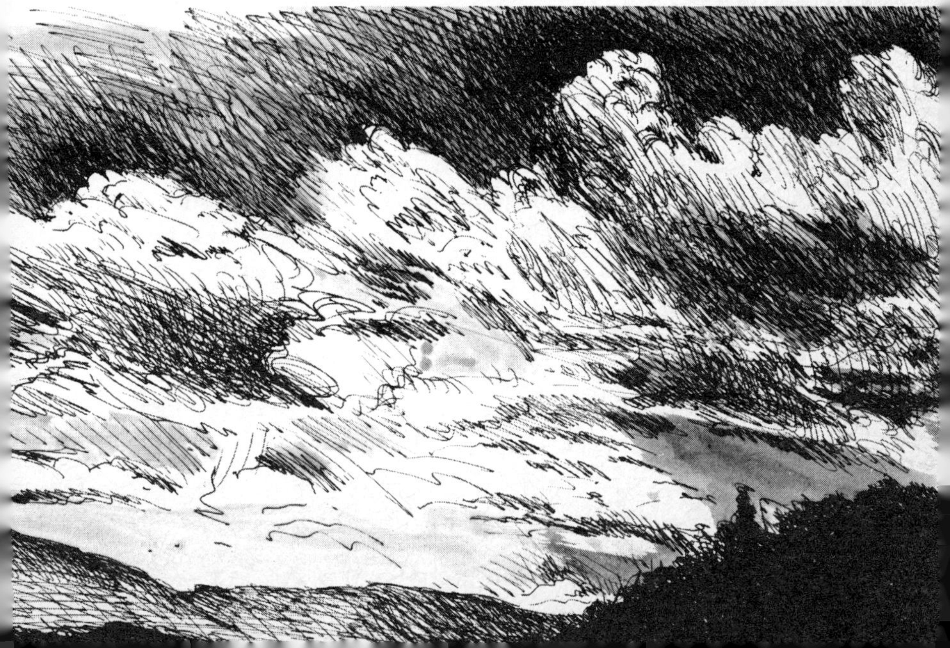

TO FOLLOW THE MACROBIOTIC WAY OF LIFE means recognition of the spiritual dimension and, consequently, the purposeful involvement in some kind of spiritual growth. That the same is true for those who profess and call themselves Christians should be too obvious to require elaboration. Since macrobiotics is not a religion there is no single form of prayer, meditation, or spiritual discipline recommended. That choice is left to the individual. To overlook the importance of inner growth and to follow other macrobiotic dietary and way of life suggestions does not produce a macrobiotic but simply a person who eats macrobiotically. There is an enormous difference between the two, although, sooner or later any person following the macrobiotic diet inevitably recognizes the need for attention to inner growth. Such recognition would evolve as balance is established and memory of human origins is restored. In macrobiotic literature the subject of spiritual growth is called self-reflection.

The reason that such a secular sounding category implies awareness of things spiritual is found in the meaning of the word "self." Michio Kushi offers the following definition:

> Self-reflection is to use our own higher consciousness to observe, review, examine and judge our thoughts and behavior which are motivated by our lower consciousness.[1]

In answering the question, "in self-reflection who is the self doing the reflecting and who is the self reflected?" we encounter the essence of any spiritual work. Indeed, pursuing that very question is a spiritual discipline in its own right. Questions found in widely scattered disciplines range from "Know thyself!" to Ramana Maharshi's *vichara,* "Who am I?" to Zen meditation on the question, "Who is it that hears?"

In his excellent book, *Basic Macrobiotics*, Herman Aihara suggests that to overcome the fear of illness one must make the commitment, "I am going to cure my disease." In elaborating this point he gives an interesting interpretation of the nature of self:

> The commitment you make doesn't come from yourself, it comes from outside yourself, from the "big Self" or universal Self. There is no fear involved—only a calm, clear understanding. Commitment, then, is made by the big Self, and the small self (what you normally identify with, the ego or conscious mind) is only a receiver. The measure of your success or defeat in life depends on the clarity of your understanding that you are part of the larger Self. If your perception of this fact is very clear you can overcome any difficulty. All difficulties, whether cancer or an uncontrollable urge to eat ice cream, are rooted in one's identifying with the small self and not the Self.[2]

Here we have a connection made between "self" and the seven principles: Aihara's "big Self" is that which recognizes its origin in the infinite one. The big Self "comes from outside yourself," and, therefore, manifests as the supreme level of judgment. In *The New English Bible* the word usually translated "soul" is translated "self" in Matthew 16:25, 26 and renders Jesus' teaching as particularly interesting in this discussion:

> Jesus then said to his disciples, "If anyone wishes to be a follower of mine he must leave self behind; he must take up his cross and come with me. Whoever cares for his own safety is lost; but if a man will let himself be lost for my sake, he will find his true self. What will a man gain by winning the whole world, at the cost of his true self? Or what can he give that will buy that self back?

Admittedly, the word in question translated "true self" is a difficult one because of the Old Testament use of "soul" as life principle. Also, the Greek influence on the New Testament elevated the word to something more than a derivative of the word for breath. But the translation quoted above captures the essential multidimensional nature of identity. There is this "big Self" one with all that is, an unchanging identity which, because it is not ephemeral, can be called the "true self." There is also that dimension in human nature which, in Herman Aihara's words, "you normally identify with" and which *does* change—"I'm a child. I'm a student. I'm young. I'm middle aged. I am well dressed. I am in rags. I am happy. I am sad." It is that small self which macrobiotics and Christianity call us to leave behind as we identify our great or true self with the eternal and infinite. The Christian would add, "through Jesus Christ our Lord," but the effect on consciousness is the same. Being born again is being born into awareness of our true identity, like discovering that we are children of the reigning king and queen but, as toddlers, had wandered away from the castle and were lost.

Self-reflection is the natural result of the practice of awareness as discussed in Chapter 11. There is no way for what Michio Kushi calls the "high consciousness" to be accessible without awareness and reflection on our lives from the perspective of increasingly higher levels of judgment until the reflection comes from the level of supreme judgment, from the true self. To expect that one will immediately be able to reflect from the big Self may be a rather big expectation. However, to use the seven levels of judgment model, it is possible to reflect from any level of judgment upon any of the lower levels. Self-reflection is self reinforcing and, therefore, fosters access to higher and higher levels. This is apparent if we look at the point Herman Aihara was making in his big Self—little self analysis, "How to Overcome the Fear of Illness." I have known people who were terrified by their diseases. Imagine what a reward it would be to be free of this fear while the difficulty is still manifesting rather than having to wait for the cessation of symptoms. The choice is obvious to all but the deeply committed masochist. If there has been no realization of the higher self, each difficulty brings the feeling of being a chip caught in a whirlpool waiting for fortuitous extrication by some errant gust of wind or benign eddy. The world is filled with those who feel so trapped.

Self-reflection offers an option, the core of which is responsibility and positive personal power. Those who perceive themselves trapped are also those who feel powerless. There is no one more trapped, physically, than a person in prison. Dietrich Bonhoeffer was a prisoner of the Nazi's. Yet, through self-reflection he came to realize that it was the jailer who had to make his regular appointed rounds who was really trapped, while Bonhoeffer was free to be who he was although behind bars. He took his own reality into the hands of his own consciousness. There are many whose spirits have soared while their bodies were incarcerated. Most of Paul's letters were written while he was being held prisoner. Bahá'u'lláh, the late 19th Century Persian, received his inspiration and dictated the literature upon which the Bahá'í faith is built while he was in prison. These people did not identify with the small self!

The process of self-reflection begins with awareness of its possibility. This possibility can be experienced in the act of describing a difficult situation. In crisis counseling it is often apparent that the level of consciousness at which a difficulty is being experienced is not the level from which the description of the difficulty is made. The totally distraught person who enters the office for counseling will, in time, offer rather dispassionate descriptions of the problem which produced the turmoil with words like, "I wish I could get a grip on myself because I know how much this is messing me up!" This is a level of self-reflection in which a bigger self is reflecting on a smaller self. At that point it is fruitful to ask, "who is the one who can 'get a grip' and who is being messed up?" Whoever it is that can "get a grip" is the one with whom we seek increasing identification, because this is the one who can see clearly enough to postulate the solution of establishing conditions which allow one to "get a grip." Actually, the dimension of the whole self which needs to be grasped is not that part having the problem but the consciousness which perceives the possibility of a solution—the bigger self.

Once awareness has come, and the watchman or witness is able to report, action must be taken. In the words of the Epistle of

James, "Be doers of the word and not hearers only, deceiving yourselves," (James 1:22). There is deception in hearing the report and not acting upon it. By so doing, the small self is deceived into thinking that it is the highest self. It has not recognized the validity of the report of the witness whose perspective encompasses greater territory. The person who has climbed the tree can see the bus coming long before those standing on the ground, who pessimistically assure each other it will never arrive. When the one up the tree shouts, "Here it comes!" those below begin gathering their belongings and getting their tickets ready. To ignore the report from the higher perspective is a sure way to miss the bus.

It is the response to the report, the doing, which occupies our interest for the remainder of this chapter. What is done in response to the report depends upon the nature of the report, but we live in an age where the need to do something to foster identity with the highest self is enormous, judging by the number of possibilities offered. The aptly named "self-help" movements offer up a varied platter from which to choose: EST, ARICA, Ekankar, Biofeedback, Dream Work, Psychosynthesis, Wholemind, Out of Body Training, Yogas: Ashtanga, Karma, Iyengar, Kripalu, Raja, Bhakti, Hatha, Krya, *et al.* In addition to the recognized religions of the world there are a variety of meditation techniques: TM, Zen koan, sitting, walking, running, standing on the head, listening to the inner sound current, listening to the outer sound current, awareness or insight, chaotic, cycling the light, staring at the light, visualization, watching the breath, chanting either Christian arrow prayers or a mantra, a meaningless word, or a meaningful word, doing Japa, saying a rosary. There is the universal language of music, "singing and making melody to the Lord with all your heart," (Ephesians 5:19). This practice is called "singing Bhajans" in India. There is dancing, too: Sufi, modern, under colored lights of specific wave lengths, in the sun, to the sun, under the moon, in the dark, as a prelude to meditation or until the dancer drops from exhaustion. Needless to say this is only a partial list, and the humor which must attend such a catalogue points up an important truth about spiritual growth—it is absolutely personal, unique, and should be approached with a sense of freedom.

Many spiritual growth disciplines, especially those associated with world religions, have some aspect of group experience or corporate worship. "Private prayer," as it is called in Christianity, may partake of some of the forms of group prayer, but must not be limited by or measured against the ritual and ceremony of corporate worship. The instruction offered by Jesus is: "When you pray, go into your room and shut the door and pray to your father . . ." (Matthew 6:6). Similarly, he suggests that the private acts of prayer and fasting not be attended by some outward display difficult to separate from ego gratification or aggrandizement of the little self: "When you fast, do not look like the hypocrites, for they disfigure their faces that they may be seen by men," (Matthew 6:16). What goes on as the result of each person's self-reflection is no one else's business except, perhaps, a spiritual director whose experience and insight is sought. In this matter pure pragmatism holds: does it feel right, does it seem to help, and is it edifying? For some it is standing on their heads while chanting, for others it is kneeling, sitting crosslegged, or lying flat on the back. The latter position was discovered by Fr. Bernard Basset at a seminar on relaxation and its virtues are recounted in his book, *Let's Start Praying Again.*[3] His slender volume is filled with worthwhile suggestions. When deciding on a path of private prayer the principle, No Two Things are Identical, is of foremost consideration. The question is: What is balancing for your unique need?

Prayer creates the path of our return to the infinite one. When Paul says, "Pray without ceasing," (1 Thessalonians 5:17), he is not just holding out a goal toward which to strive. He means it. As Aelred Squire points out so well:

> Now it must be regarded as very significant that not a single

> Christian writer of antiquity, no matter how heretical, ever thought of interpreting these commands to pray always as though they could be taken metaphorically.[4]

It was this piece of scripture which drove the subject of the book *The Pilgrim* on his quest for a way to fulfill Paul's admonition. He found ceaseless repetition of the Jesus Prayer—Lord Jesus Christ, have mercy upon me—to be the goal of his search. In this case "prayer" actually began as a prayer, but, if prayer is to be ceaseless, it must be an activity which is entered into at such a deep level of being that other, surface activities can be carried on without losing the state of consciousness which represents underlying awareness of that deep level. Prayer may have little to do with prayers. Perhaps we should paraphrase Paul with the words, "Be prayerful without ceasing." A prayerful attitude is the foundation on which ceaseless prayer can be built. Indeed, the pilgram found that in time his mantra descended from head to heart and was constantly being said by the heart. It became a prayer of the heart even while he was asleep. Prayers, whether ready-made or original, should be expressions of prayerfulness and lead us on into further prayerfulness. With this in mind it is apparent that prayers are sometimes prayer, sometimes not. Compared with the popular notion of prayer as a set verbal ritual this definition allows for inclusion of any ongoing self reflective process in the category of prayer, even if it has descended to an involuntary depth. Therefore, whatever is being done with grateful awareness is prayer.

There is no way to separate preparation for spiritual growth, or evolution of consciousness, from the process itself. Tilling the soil in preparation for planting is gardening just as much as the sowing of the seeds. Macrobiotic practice is also both preparation and actualization of the expansion of consciousness toward realization of true identity. In awareness of the manifestation of the universal truths described by the seven principles, in the application of the laws of change to the selection, preparation and grateful consumption of food, in the willingness to choose the upward path or the way of life, the miasma of death which casts its pall on contemporary consciousness is dispelled. As the clear light dawns and moves to its zenith, revealing our source, sustenance, and substance as that very light, shadows of mortality shorten and disappear. Once we are on the way there is no possibility of separating the path from the goal. Our awareness, self-reflection and choice of action are preparing, embarking, travelling, and arriving. It is all one trip. Isaiah described the process in these words:

> A voice cries: "In the wilderness prepare the way of the Lord, make straight in the desert a highway for our God. Every valley shall be lifted up, and every mountain and hill be made low; the uneven ground shall become level, and the rough places a plain. And the glory of the Lord shall be revealed, and all flesh shall see it together, for the mouth of the Lord has spoken." (Isaiah 40:3–5)

There are several practices which I have found to be especially beneficial. Each of us, I am sure, would have a different list. The following is offered with the assurance that the methods have worked for me at various times and seasons of my life.

The postures of Hatha Yoga seem to be preparatory in that they offer a way to loosen up physical tightness and produce a state of relaxation. Once loosened up and relaxed we can get down to what is usually thought of as the real thing. The Hatha postures *are* the real thing. J. M. Dechanet, in his book, *Christian Yoga,*[5] lays to rest qualms which might arise in the minds of those whose Christianity is so exclusive that they might hesitate to practice a discipline whose roots lie in another religion. Such hesitation is very real in some quarters, but the benefits of this gentle practice prove what should be obvious: there is no such thing as a Hindu body, a Buddhist body, or a Christian body. Humans seeking the light have evolved methods which enable revelation of that light and those methods are appropriate for others regardless of theological systems. Hatha postures also form a bridge between the dimensions of body and spirit by providing an external application of the progression toward flexibility fostered by following macrobiotic dietary suggestions. Chaotic food patterns, which are both the cause and the result of personal and social chaos, produce inflexibility on all levels. To be inflexible in this ever-changing universe is to fly flagrantly in the face of reality. Something has to give. This ever-changing universe does not stop changing to accommodate to the misperception of a static reality. What gives and even breaks is mental, physical, and spiritual health. Stretch your muscles. Stretch your mind. Stretch your dreams and expectations until they encompass their true identity in infinity.[6]

Included in the Hatha yoga discipline is the practice of pranayama or balancing of the subtle energies which find expression in the breath. The practice of alternating nostrils in breathing by physically prevénting the air from entering has a remarkably balancing effect. This practice has been used since the time of Gregory Palamas, in the early 14 Century, by the Hesychasts of the Greek Orthodox Church. For almost six hundred years Hatha practice has been a recognized part of Christian spiritual development.

The power of autosuggestion is enormous. Words we say are like seeds sown, and they grow in the fertile soil of our subconscious minds to bear fruit—sometimes when we least expect it. Paul's admonition to the Philippians recognizes the power of thought:

> And now, my friends, all that is true, all that is noble, all that is just and pure, all that is lovable and gracious, whatever is excellent and admirable—fill your thoughts with these things, (Philippians 4:8).

This suggestion is a very serious one. It is not the idle musing of someone obsessively religious. Thoughts of worry, anger, fear, retribution all sow seeds. They are prayers for the very scenario to manifest. Such thoughts also indicate that the thinker has some distance to go before fully grasping the meaning of the seven principles. If thought seeds can be sown, they can be controlled. Positive thoughts can replace negative ones. These positive thoughts are called affirmations, arrow prayers, or declarations. Said out loud, they can have a powerful effect deep in one's being. Repeated silently they can keep the mind fixed on the light side of complementary opposites.

Strictly speaking, affirmations and arrow prayers are not the same, but their effect is similar. The Jesus Prayer, so much loved by the Eastern church, is an example of the combination of a positive thought with a general petition for mercy. In truth, there is nothing but mercy offered by the divine economy. Especially in repetitive prayer, the tendency to ask for specifics should be avoided. It is not out task to write the agenda for reality but to celebrate it as it manifests and to have faith in the justice of whatever comes.

The affirmation, then, should be short, simple, and non specific. A petition for guidance, light, or wholeness is to be preferred. For instance, healing may come as understanding rather than as the immediate reversal of a physical condition. The affirmation of Emile Coué, "Every day in every way I am getting better and better," is a tremendously effective statement. It recognizes the reality of moment to moment change, that the person, ""I," is part of that change, and that the change is for the better or that justice is being done, whatever that might be for each person. I recommend this particular affirmation most highly, along with the technique for its use which Coué suggests. Some counting device—a string with twenty knots tied in it, or twenty beads on a chain—is used. As one is falling asleep and is in that hypnogogic state known to provide access to deep parts of the being, the affirmation is said twenty times. The first time, equal emphasis is placed on each word or phrase, but during successive recitations each part is emphasized in turn. "*Day by day* in every way . . ." is followed by, "Day by day *in every way* . . ." and then, "Day by day in every way *I am* getting . . ." and so on. This procedure is repeated immediately upon waking. I found the latter time to be extremely difficult for me, but the purpose of suggesting it is that it provides a similar state of consciousness to the moment of falling asleep.

Do you feel silly at first sounding like *The Little Engine that Could,* saying the same thing over and over? Yes. Does it work? Yes. Compose some affirmations for your own use. Remember to make them short, simple, positive, and general. Say them as Emile Coué suggests, or all day long, or whenever you think of it. You will be surprised at two things: how difficult it is at first to remember to do it, and how effective the practice is once it is established. Affirmations are a living-out of Paul's advice to the Colossians, "Set your minds on things that are above," (3:2). They are a way to "make in the desert a highway for our God."

Visualization, or "active imagination," as Gerald Jampolsky calls it in *Love is Letting go of Fear,* uses pictures instead of words as the vehicle of expression. This form of prayerfulness is ancient and universal. Visualization is used by anyone who creates in order to build a thought form of that thing which will be created. Artists use visualization to see the statue awaiting to be revealed within the stone, the picture yet to be put on canvas. Visual images transcend the barriers of language. Each *is* worth a thousand words.

The power of visualization has achieved media attention recently in the work of Carl Simonton and Stephanie Matthews-Simonton.[7] They have had success with cancer patients who have used imagery specific to their particular form of disease. The natural immune system is visualized as overcoming the cancer cells in an interesting variety of civil war. Visualization is only one part of the Simonton approach, which is wholistic, but it is the centerpiece; and it is effective. The body at war with itself appeals to the popular image of cancer as invader. Therefore, the predisposition for such imagery is in place for most people. However, the nature of this particular visualization is not consonant with macrobiotic understanding. Since antagonisms are ever-changing, complementary, equi-proportioned, unique, finite manifestations of one infinity (that covers all seven principles!), war is an inappropriate image. War, battles, and fights are only seen as appropriate by someone trapped in dualism who considers antagonisms as nothing more than antagonisms—good/bad, we/they, this/that, black/white. Such an understanding fails to comprehend the complementarity realized in macrobiotic philosophy. The cancer is there as the final stage in a whole system of unheeded warnings, the lack of awareness of which has necessitated such an extreme reminder. That the reminder has finally been heard should be cause for gratitude, not for the beginning of war with the messenger. When it is demonstrated that the message has been heard, and is being acted upon according to the laws of change, the messenger will go away. Cancer *is* a tenacious messenger because it is such an extreme condition, but it brings its reminder only to a certain person in a certain state. Change the person sufficiently and the messenger will seek someone to whom the message is more appropriate.

The Simontons have achieved success because they offer the possibility of active, personal responsibility in the cure, as well as because their total approach is wholistic. If entered into with enthusiasm, Simonton visualization can result in a new person. Visualization only can be done by the visualizer. Personal responsibility for one's condition is the key and visualization is an excellent way to exercise that responsibility.

Shakti Gawain has written a very popular little book entitled, *Creative Visualization.*[8] She offers a multitude of excellent suggestions for visual meditations around a variety of themes.

Paul reveals a meditation technique to his Corinthian friends when he confesses that he did not use "fine words," but, "I resolved that while I was with you I would think of nothing but Jesus Christ—Christ nailed to the cross," (1 Corinthians 2:2). This particular image has an interesting parallel in the writings of George Ohsawa who offers the following definition: "Meditation is nothing more than the visualization of the cross in all situations, at every level and at every step."[9] In fairness to this comparison it should be pointed out that Ohsawa would have agreed with Huston Smith's assessment of the cross as the

"Western yin-yang." Thus, ceaseless meditation on the cross is, for Ohsawa, constant recognition of the interplay of these complementary forces. Since yin/yang arises as the first act of creation, awareness of all phenomena as resulting from this basis places the consciousness very close to awareness of the infinite One from whom yin and yang proceed. This means that awareness is rooted in the "higher self," and the reflection of the lower self is seen in a mirror free from the distortions produced by lower levels of judgment.

Prayers are a very powerful means of aligning all levels of being with divine will or the order of the universe. When prayers are also prayer, or what Teresa of Avila calls "genuine devotion," the effect is immediate and total. However, even when prayers are a rote ritual an effect is produced over time which may startle the nominal believer. This fact was brought home to me when I suggested to a person who did not believe in prayer that he pray regularly as if he *did* believe. We worked out a schedule for prayers three times a day and the use of an affirmation. In a week his prayers had turned to prayer. The particular pastoral problem which had brought him to my office was well on the way to resolution.

This particular instance points out the power of *non credo*. The nonbeliever was not about to take anyone's word about the power of saying prayers. He discovered by the convincing power of personal experience what could not be communicated to him solely on the basis of trusting the validity of someone else's report. His faith became "owned." He is to be commended because he possessed a trusting spirit; he was game to give it a sincere try. Such an attitude is not always easy to find. Many people who feel stuck in their problems are experiencing the result of deep inflexibility which prevents their openness to new avenues of approach. As we have seen, the quality of clinging, or "stuckness," is not appropriate to the mode of expression which typifies life in the Kingdom. Following the macrobiotic way of life promotes flexibility. For this reason food prepared according to macrobiotic guidelines is referred to as *shōjin ryōri*—spiritual development cuisine.

There are suggestions for prayers, said or sung, in all religions. In corporate worship an atmosphere conducive to genuine devotion is created, and a power to transform prayers to prayer is generated. The difference between private prayer and corporate worship is the same as that between eating alone or dining with friends. One should not eat alone all the time. Take advantage of the power of presence which occurs "where two or three are gathered together," (Matthew 18:20).

Nicolas Herman, a 17 Century Carmelite monk known as Brother Lawrence, was widely recognized for his high spiritual development. He was a ponderous and clumsy man whose first choice of positions at the monastery would not have been the kitchen. He worked in the kitchen, however, for most of his many years with the Carmelite order. Whether by inspiration, coincidence, or good luck, he was blessed in having hit upon the heart of the practice of self-reflection. He was able to so efface his moment to moment identification with lower judgment levels that his consciousness was rooted in his highest self—God within. He called his spiritual path "the practice of the presence of God."[10] The highest self is the infinite one within. There was no way for Brother Lawrence, in his humility, to identify his *persona* with this self and so he perceived this self to be someone other than his lower self. Thus, his description of this compellingly simple practice is as follows:

> I keep myself retired with Him in the very center of my soul as much as I can; and while I am so with Him I fear nothing.
>
> I continued some years applying my mind carefully . . . to *the presence of God,* whom I considered always as with me, often as in me.
>
> We need only to recognize God intimately present with us, and to address ourselves to Him every moment.

At times he would slip in consciousness and become aware that his mind was no longer "in the presence of the Lord." When this occured he would bring his awareness back to the realization of God's presence without great concern, recognizing that forgiveness is divine. With regard to the mind he advises:

> If it sometimes wanders and withdraws itself from Him, do not much disquiet yourself for that: trouble and disquiet serve rather to distract the mind than to recall it; the will must bring it back in tranquillity.

Brother Lawrence's interviewer, whose comments are included in editions of *The Practice of The Presence of God,* rightly observes, "His view of prayer was nothing else but a sense of the Presence of God." For this monk, then, prayerfulness was an everpresent state. He truly prayed "without ceasing." This fact is borne out in his belief that "it was a great delusion to think that the times of prayer ought to differ from other times."

Brother Lawrence travelled the high road from the day of his conversion at the age of eighteen when he realized the hopefulness implicit in the eternal law of change:

> In the winter, seeing a tree stripped of its leaves, and considering that within a little time the leaves would be renewed, and after that the flowers and fruit appear, he received a high view of the providence and power of God, which has never since been effaced from his soul.

Is not the "high view" at the heart of the issue for us all? From this view one is able to perceive and be grateful for both the unity and the necessity of the world of this and that. The high road which affords this view is the one we have sought to follow in the preceding pages, seeking the wisdom of past and present fellow travellers, and pointing to milestones and road signs along the way. Much to the detriment of the planet earth and all of her creatures, the high road in our time is not crowded with pilgrims.

Nonetheless, it is a highway in the desert for our God; it is the road of the kingdom; it is the way of life.

> I call heaven and earth to witness against you this day, that I have set before you life and death, blessing and curse; therefore choose life, that you and your descendants may live, loving the Lord your God, obeying his voice, and cleaving to him; for that means life to you and length of days. . . . (Deuteronomy 30: 19, 20a)

[1] Kushi, *Book of Macrobiotics,* p. 164.
[2] Aihara, *Basic Macrobiotics,* p. 49.
[3] Basset, *Let's Sart Praying Again,* Herder and Herder, 1972.
[4] Squire, *Asking The Fathers,* pp. 140, 141.
[5] Dechanet, *Christian Yoga,* Harper and Row, 1960.
[6] In addition to the above volume, *Integral Yoga Hatha,* by Swami Satchidananda, Holt, Rinehart and Winston, 1970, is one of the best, with clear pictures and text. However, classes are recommended since it is difficult to capture the pace and spirit of yoga practice in print. Classes also help to prevent improper practice from becoming habit.
[7] Simonton, Matthews-Simonton, and Creighton, *Getting Well Again,* Tarcher, 1978.
[8] Shakti Gawain, *Creative Visualization,* Bantam, 1978.
[9] Ohsawa, *Jack and Mitie in The West,* p. 212.
[10] *Brother Lawrence, The Practice of The Presence of God,* All quotes from Brother Lawrence are from this Forward Movement Publications pamphlet, available from the publisher at very modest cost, 412 Sycamore St., Cincinnati, Ohio 45202.

Bibliography

Aihara, Herman. *Seven Basic Macrobiotic Principles.* Magalia, CA: The Grain and Salt Society

———. *Learning from Salmon,* Oroville, CA: G.O.M.F., 1980

———. *Basic Macrobiotics,* Tokyo: Japan Publications., 1985

Basset, Bernard. *Let's Start Praying Again.* New York: Herder and Herder, 1972

Beare, Francis W. *The Earliest Records of Jesus.* New York: Abingdon, 1972

———. *St. Paul and His Letters.* New York: Abingdon, 1962

Bettenson, Henry. *Documents of the Christian Church.* New York: Oxford University Press, 1963

Blakney, Raymond B., Trans. *Meister Eckhart: A Modern Translation.* New York: Harper & Row, 1941

Bouquet, A. C. *Sacred Books of The World.* London: Penguin Books, 1953

———. *Everyday Life in New Testament Times.* New York: Scribner, 1954

Brown, Raymond E. *The Community of The Beloved Disciple.* New York: Paulist, 1979

Breech, James. *The Silence of Jesus.* Philadelphia: Fortress Press, 1983

Buchwald, Art. *Down The Seine and Up The Potomac.* New York: G. P. Putnam's Sons, 1956–1977

Cady, H. Emilie. *Lessons in Truth.* Unity Village, MO: Unity Books

Canty, Jerome. *Sounding The Sacred Conch.* Boulder, CO: Amazeing Books, 1981

Capra, Fritjof. *The Turning Point.* New York: Simon and Schuster, 1982

Chesterton, G. K. *St. Francis of Assisi.* Garden City, N.Y.: Image Books, Doubleday, 1957

Cousins, Norman. *Anatomy of an Illness.* New York: W. W. Norton, 1979

Cox, Harvey. *Religion in The Secular City*. New York: Simon and Schuster, 1984
Daniel-Rops, Henri. *Daily Life in The Time of Jesus*. New York: Hawthorn Books, 1962
Davies, Paul. *God and The New Physics*. New York: Simon and Schuster, 1983
Dechanet, J. M. *Christian Yoga*. New York: Harper and Row, 1960
De Chardin, Teilhard. *The Divine Milieu. New York: Harper and* Row, 1960
Dodd, C. H. *The Apostolic Preaching*. New York: Harper & Bros, 1970
Drake, Katia and Jonathan. *Natural Birth Control*. Wellingborough, England: Thorsons, 1984
Dufty, William. *You are All Sanpaku*. Secaucus, N.J.: Citadel, 1965
Dulles, Avery. *Models of Revelation*. Garden City, N.Y.: Doubleday, 1983
Esko, Edward and Wendy. *Macrobiotic Cooking for Everyone*. Tokyo and New York: Japan Publications, 1980
Feldenkrais, Moshe. *Awareness Through Movement*. New York: Harper and Row, 1972
———. *The Elusive Obvious*. M. Feldenkrais, 1981
Fox, Matthew. *Original Blessing*. Santa Fe: Bear & Co., 1983
Goldberg, Philip. *The Intuitive Edge*. Los Angeles: Jeremy Tarcher, 1983
Goldstein, Joseph. *The Experience of Insight*. Boston: Shambhala, 1983
Grant, Michael. *Jesus, an Historian's Review of The Gospels*. New York: Charles Scribner's Sons, 1977
Guillaumont, A., *et al.* Tr. *The Gospel According to Thomas*. New York: Harper and Row, 1959
Hick, John. *God Has Many Names*. New York: Macmillan, 1980
———, *Evil and The God of Love*. New York: Harper and Row, 1966
———. *Death and Eternal Life*. New York: Harper & Row, 1976
Holy Bible, Revised Standard Version. New York: Thomas Nelson and Sons, 1957
Hunter, Archibald M. *Paul and His Predecessors*. Philadelphia: The Westminster Press, 1961
James, Fleming. *Personalities of The Old Testament*. New York: Charles Scribner, 1939

Jampolsky, Gerald G. *Love is Letting Go of Fear*. Berkeley, CA: Celestial Arts, 1979
Kervran, Louis C. *Biological Transmutations*. Brooklyn: Swan House, 1972
Kushi, Michio. *The Book of Macrobiotics*. Tokyo and New York: Japan Publications, 1977
———. *The Macrobiotic Way*. Avery: Wayne, N. J., 1985
———. *Natural Healing Through Macrobiotics*. Tokyo and New York: Japan Publications, 1978
Lemisch, Jessie L., *Benjamin Franklin*. New York: The New American Library, 1961
Leon-Portilla, Miguel, *Native MesoAmerican Spirituality*. New York: Paulist Press, 1980
Levine, Stephen. *A Gradual Awakening*. Garden City, N.Y.: Doubleday, 1979
Main, Dom John. *Talks on Meditation*. Montreal: The Benedictine Community, 1979
MacLeod, Fiona. *The Isle of Dreams*. Portland, ME.: Thomas B. Mosher, 1905
Maureau, Paul M. *The Massardis Saga*. Woolwich, ME: TBW Books, 1984
Merton, Thomas. *The Way of Chuang Tzu*. New York: New Directions, 1969
———. *Zen and The Birds of Appetite*. New York: New Directions, 1968
Moltmann, Jurgen. *Theology of Hope*. Edinburgh: T. & A. Constable, 1967
Moss, Claude B. *The Christian Faith*. New York: Morehouse-Gorham, 1957
Muramoto, Naboru. *Healing Ourselves*. New York: Avon Books, 1973
New English Bible. New York: Oxford University Press, 1976
Nouwen, Henri J. M. *Pray to Live*. Notre Dame: Fides, 1972
Ohsawa, George. *The Book of Judgment*. Oroville, CA: George Ohsawa Macrobiotic Found, 1980
———. *Guidebook for Living*. Los Angeles: GOMF, 1967
———. *Macrobiotics: An Invitation to Health and Happiness*. Oroville, CA: George Ohsawa Macrobiotic Foundation, 1978
———. *The Unique Principle*. Oroville, CA: GOMF, 1976

———. *Zen Macrobiotics*. Los Angeles: George Ohsawa Macrobiotic Foundation, 1965

Palmer, G. E. H., ed. *The Philokalia, Vol. 1*. Boston: Faber and Faber, 1979

———. *The Philokalia, Vol. 2*. Boston: Faber and Faber, 1981

Peck, M. Scott. *The Road Less Traveled*. New York: Simon and Schuster, 1978

Prestige, G. L. *Fathers and Heretics*. London: S.P.C.K., 1954

Purtill, Richard L. *C. S. Lewis's Case for the Christian Faith*. New York: Harper and Row, 1981

Rivers, Jerry M., *et al. Planning Meals that Lower Cancer Risk: A Reference Guide*. Washington: American Institute for Cancer Research, 1984

Robinson, John A. T., *In The End God*. New York: Harper and Row, 1968

Satchidananda, Yogiraj Sri Swami. *Integral Yoga Hatha*. New York: Holt, Rinehart, & Winston, 1970

Schumacher, E. F., *Small is Beautiful*. New York: Harper and Row, 1975

Simcox, Carroll E. *A Treasury of Quotations on Christian Themes*. New York: Seabury, 1975

Simonton, L. Carl, Matthews-Simonton, Stephanie, Creighton, James. *Getting Well Again*. Los Angeles: Tarcher, 1978

Singh, Tara. *Gratefulness*. Los Angeles: Foundation for Life Action, 1981

Smith, Huston. *Forgotten Truth*. New York: Harper and Row, 1976

Spong, John Shelby. *This Hebrew Lord*. New York: Seabury, 1974

Squire, Aelred. *Asking The Fathers*. New York: Morehouse Barlow, 1973

Steindl-Rast, Bro David. *Gratefulness, The Heart of Prayer*. New York: Paulist Press, 1984

Symans, Gilbert P., Ed. *Brother Lawrence, The Practice of The pressence of God*. Cincinnati: Forward Movement

Taylor, John V. *The Go-Between God*. London: SCM, 1972

Thornton, Martin. *Spiritual Direction*. Boston: Cowley Publications, 1984

Tooker, Elisabeth, Ed. *Native North American Spirituality of The Eastern Woodlands*. New York: Paulist Press, 1979

Toynbee, Arnold. *A Study of History*. New York: Oxford University Press, 1972

Trumbull, H. Clay. *Blood Covenant*. New York: Charles Scribner, 1885

Veith, Ilza. *The Yellow Emperor's Classic of Internal Medicine*. Los Angeles: University of California Press, 1949

Ward, Benedicta. *The Desert Christian*. New York: Macmillan, 1975

Whiston, William. *The Works of Flavius Josephus*. Philadelphia: International Press

Wilkinson, L. P. *Virgil, The Georgics*. New York: Penguin, 1982

Biblical Reference Index

Old Testament

New Testament

General Index